In Search of

20/20

In Search of

20/20

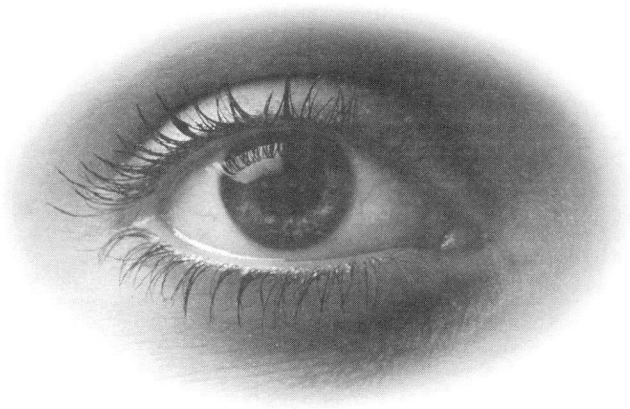

Everything You Need to Know About

Laser Eye Surgery

Arun Lakra M.D. **Howard V. Gimbel** M.D.

GES

Canadian Cataloguing in Publication Data

Lakra, Arun, 1966-
In Search of 20/20

Includes index.

1...Eye-Refractive errors--Treatment--Popular works. 2.Eye-
-Laser surgery--Popular works.   I. Gimbel, Howard V., 1934-
II. Title. III. Title: In search of twenty/twenty.

RE86.L34 1997   617.7'55   C97-910013-5

ISBN 0-9681756-0-0

Cover Design: Carbon Media Inc.
Illustrations: Stephanie Chamberland
Statistical Graphs: Maria Ferensowicz & Micheline Deschenes
Cartoons: Written by Arun Lakra & Illustrated by Mark Cromwell of
     The Color Club
Author Photographs: Appletree Photographic Arts, Bilodeau/Preston

Although every precaution has been taken in the preparation of this book, the publisher and
authors assume no responsibility for errors or omissions. No liability is assumed for damages
resulting from the use of the information contained herein. All product names identified in
this book are trademarks, registered trademarks and trade names of their
respective companies. No uses of any trade name are intended to convey endorsement or
other affiliation with this book.

This book is not intended to replace the recommendations of a doctor. All decisions should be
made in consultation with a physician. Any information set forth in this book is at the reader's
discretion.

Printed in Canada

For
N and D

Forever 20/20
If Vision is Love

Contents at a Glance

Contents

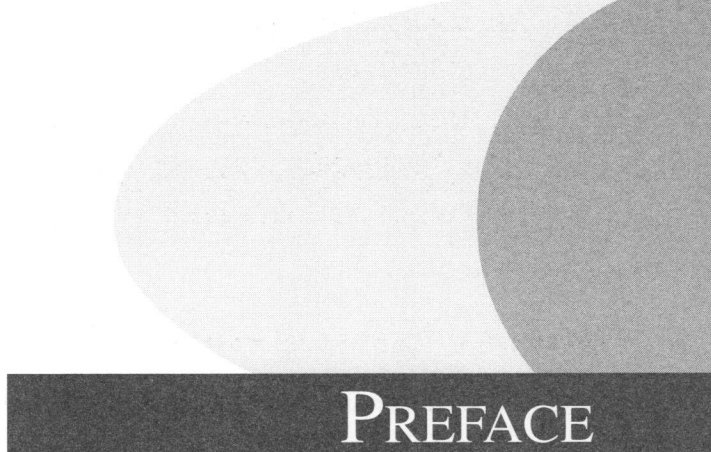

PREFACE

This book is designed to be objective, accurate, comprehensive, easy-to-read, and current.

Objectivity is the most important element. With any medical procedure, especially an elective one, there are risks and benefits, pros and cons, overexuberant optimism and unfounded fears. There are many sides, perspectives, and opinions regarding the whole question of refractive eye surgery, and it is our goal to present all of them in an unbiased fashion.

Accuracy of our facts and results has been a priority. The statistics presented are derived from two sources. The primary source is the computerized data storage and analysis system of the Gimbel Eye Centre in Calgary, Canada. This institution is one of the world leaders in the field of refractive surgery. It was there that the first Canadian PRK was peformed. In fact, since 1986, at the Gimbel Eye Centre, approximately 9000 RK, 12,000 PRK, 1000 LASIK, and 38,000 cataract extraction/lensectomy procedures have been performed. In the case of isolated procedures which have not been performed at this institution (such as Holmium LTK), data which has not been recorded there, and RK data as a whole, the results presented in this book are derived from the scientific literature. There is some degree of variability in the real world. For example, there may be a 90 percent chance of achieving 20/20 vision post-operatively at the Gimbel Eye Centre. Other surgeons at other institutions will have slightly different results. Because of this variability in refractive surgery, these statistics are presented as a guide only. The chance of obtaining a specific result depends on your eyes and your surgeon, and consequently, should be individualized.

This book is intended to be a *comprehensive* review of refractive surgery for the lay person. Still, it is impossible to include every potential risk, benefit, complication, and alternative treatment. The information contained in this book, therefore, is incomplete. Careful consideration has been given to what should be included and excluded, with relevance playing the deciding role.

It is easy to say *easy-to-read*. When dealing with a technical subject such as refractive eye surgery, however, it is easier said than done. A foundation of principles and terms are described in a sequential fashion. Although it may be tempting to jump to the more alluring laser sections immediately, this may result in some confusion. Invest a little time and effort in learning the vocabulary and understanding the principles. It will pay off.

Refractive eye surgery has been described as a tidal wave about to hit our shores. Imagine trying to take a photograph of this wave. A snapshot taken right now may appear quite different to another one shot ten seconds from now. The only thing constant about refractive eye surgery is change. Our best efforts have been devoted to bringing you up-to-the-minute, *current* information, however you should keep a lookout for new ideas and data on the horizon. The good news is that the principles will likely remain very much the same, with the specifics and the results being most susceptible to variability.

May your search for 20/20 be insightful and rewarding.

The authors

INTRODUCTION

So you're searching for 20/20. And you've heard about laser eye surgery. Maybe a friend told you about it or perhaps you saw an ad on television. Now let us go out on a limb. Somewhere, at the tip of your tongue, or at the very least at the back of your mind, there is a question. Should you have laser eye surgery? It's a very simple question, really. A yes or no question. And you've picked up this book hoping for a quick answer, so you can get back to making important decisions like what to have for dinner tonight.

Should I have laser eye surgery? Everywhere we go, people ask us this. Should I have laser eye surgery? It's a loaded question. In fact, it's an excellent question to ask, only a difficult one to answer. And although it is cleverly disguised, it really isn't a yes or no question. It's like asking someone, "Should I buy a car?"

A car. Well, do you really need a car? What about public transportation? Or bicycles or cabs? Or even walking? Can you afford a car? And what kind of car are we talking about here? A sports car or a sedan? What's more important to you, comfort or style? Speed or reliability? Are airbags really necessary? And if you're so scared of what can happen to you in a car, then maybe you shouldn't even be on the roads.

Similar issues can be raised about laser eye surgery. Do you really need it? What are the alternatives? When it comes to your eyes, what's more important to you, appearance or function? Safety or style? As you can see, there are a number of questions which need to be addressed before you're anywhere near making a decision. And everybody is different. Each person has different priorities, different expectations and goals, and importantly, different eyes. So whether you're in search of a perfect car or perfect vision, it is a decision you have to make and to live with.

With due respect to car dealers and manufacturers, we are talking about your eyes. This is serious business and you know it. There are no 100% guarantees in medicine and there is no chance of getting replacement eyes if yours are in the shop. The most important thing is to make the best decision you can.

When you are in the market for a new car, you do some research. You talk to friends and family, even car salesmen. You read consumer reports. And once you have all of the information you need, you make a decision. In car-shopping, however, you have a bit of a head start. You already know that a car has four wheels, a steering wheel, and runs on gasoline. And you also have a little perspective, knowing that brakes shouldn't be an optional accessory. Last but not least, you have the benefit of having driven a car before and also being able to test drive before you buy.

The same principles apply when considering laser eye surgery. The difference is here, you're starting from scratch. In all probability, you don't know very much about laser eye surgery. You don't know about its history, its results, its inherent risks. Chances are you don't know much about the different kinds of laser eye surgery and what is the best kind for you. Perhaps you don't even know very much about eyes in general and your eyes in particular.

You are not alone. Greater than a quarter of the population is nearsighted. An additional percentage is farsighted. It is estimated that by the year 2000, three million Americans will have had laser eye surgery. And two million more will undergo the procedure every year after that. Countless more will consider it. That means that each person like you, who endures glasses or contact lenses, is today confronted with a difficult decision. With the health of your eyes at stake, not to mention the issues of money, pain, risk, and unknown chances of success, how do you make such a decision?

That is why we are asked questions at social gatherings. Intelligent, motivated, responsible people like you are attempting to acquire all of the information they can in order to make the right decision. The problem is figuring out who to ask. You can seek the advice of people at cocktail parties, but anecdotal accounts can be misleading. You can ask your eye doctor, but that is not unlike asking a car salesman if you should buy his or her car. You can search the archives of medical literature in search of relevant, accurate, information. Buried under mountains of statistics and obscured by clouds of bias you may discover useful facts.

Or you can read on. We have attempted to compile for you a summary of everything you need to know about laser eye surgery. The information you will read is as accurate, objective, and up-to-date as possible. Some of the sections are fairly technical. That is the nature of eye surgery. Please do not be intimidated by the fancy diagrams and the difficult to pronounce terms. You will find everything surprisingly easy to understand. And that is the goal. For only if you understand your eyes and your options, will you be able to make the best possible decision. It is, after all, *your* decision.

PART
ONE

THE BASICS

1

SEEING

You don't need to be a mechanic to shop for a car. However, without the basics, you run a greater risk of selecting a lemon. When it comes to your eyes, the basics means anatomy and physics. Unfortunately, nobody, with the possible exception of anatomists and physicists, find these subjects especially exciting. The good news is that with a little perseverance, you can get a grasp of the important principles. So try to resist the temptation to jump to the laser chapters. Take a deep breath and dive in. Your patience and effort will be rewarded.

Before we can understand laser eye surgery and other treatments for vision problems, we must first learn how we see.

THE EYE AS A CAMERA

Creating a visual image is not very different from creating a photograph. It is helpful to think of the eye as a camera. Suppose you want to take a picture of an apple. In addition to a camera and an apple, you need one other element. (Hint: What does the L in LASER stand for?)

WHAT IS LIGHT?

At the risk of inducing high school physics flashbacks, we will make a *brief* digression in order to shed a little light on this question. Very simply, visible light is a very small part of the naturally occurring electromagnetic radiation spectrum. The same spectrum that brings you radio waves, television waves, and X-rays, also brings you visible light waves.

The only difference between these types of radiation is the wavelength. The specific wavelength will determine whether the radiation is visible or not, whether it is an X-ray or an FM radio wave. If the wavelength happens to coincide with a pigment in our retina, then we can see it. If the chemicals in our camera film respond to that specific frequency, then we can photograph it.

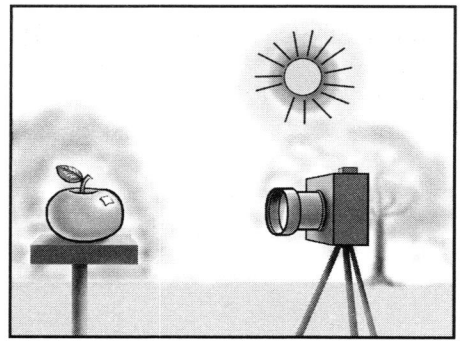

Let's return to the apple we want to photograph. Light, whether it comes from the sun, the moon, a lamp, or a flash, reaches the apple. If it is a red apple, then all of the blue and yellow wavelengths are absorbed.

The red light, however, ricochets off the surface of the apple in all directions. Some of this light comes toward our camera. This light travels through the lens and is focussed on the film. The photochemicals respond to this frequency of light and a photograph is created.

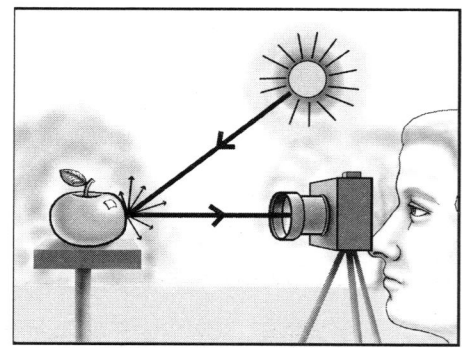

How Do We See?

Our camera, as it turns out, is a disposable one. Let's dispose of it. Who really wants a photograph of an apple anyway? Now that the camera is lying on the ground, you find yourself standing in front of the apple. Just like before, light from the sun hits the apple. Some light is absorbed and some is reflected. Now, instead of going through the camera, this light heads for your

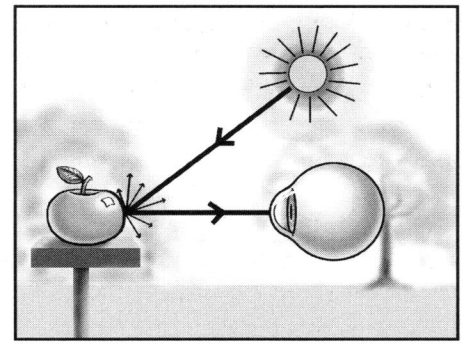

eyes. And as you stand there paralyzed with wonder, some of this light is racing toward you. Some light waves are headed in the direction of your kneecap. Other rays have targeted your left sleeve. And a few special rays, which have travelled all the way from the sun only to be rudely reflected by your apple, are destined for your eyes.

Your Eyes

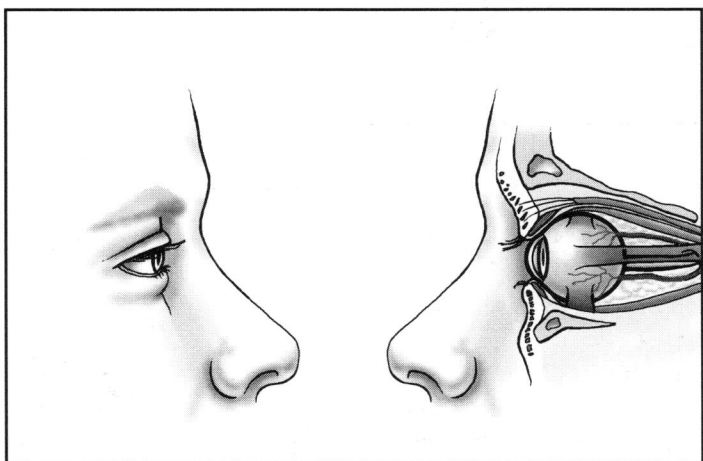

There is a lot more to the eye than meets the eye. When you look in the mirror, what you see is only the tip of the iceberg. The mirror reveals a reciprocal image with the skin and bones removed, demonstrating the entire length of the eyeball.

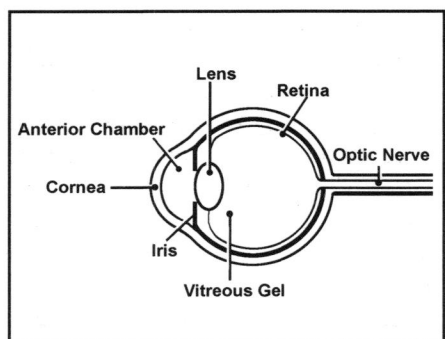

The average eyeball, or *globe*, is approximately 22 millimetres or about 7/8th of an inch long. If we were to cut it lengthwise, we would see this cross-section.

The eye is made up of many components, a few of which play an important role in vision. In our analogy, the *cornea* of the eye is the camera lens, the *pupil* is the aperture, and the *retina* is the film.

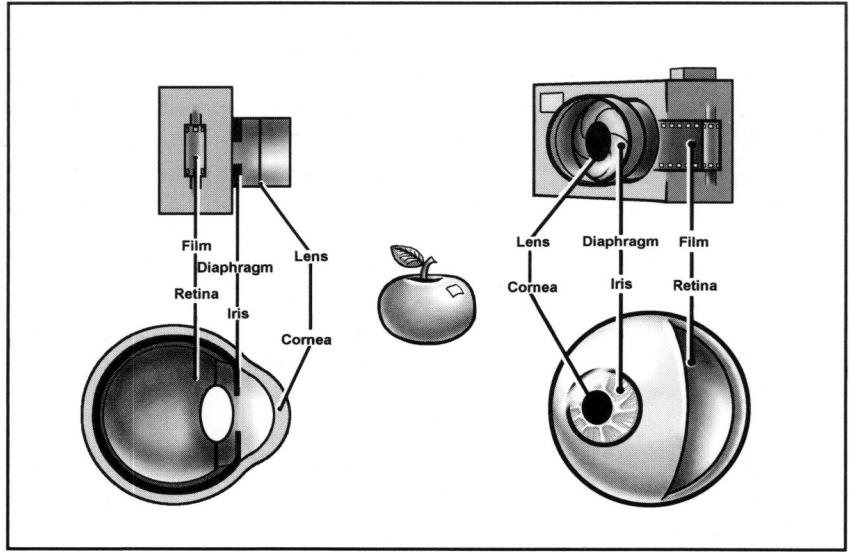

The Cornea

Anatomy: The cornea is a transparent dome which consists of several distinct layers. The *epithelium* is the outermost layer which is comprised of several layers of cells. It is similar to the epidermis of the skin, only the tough

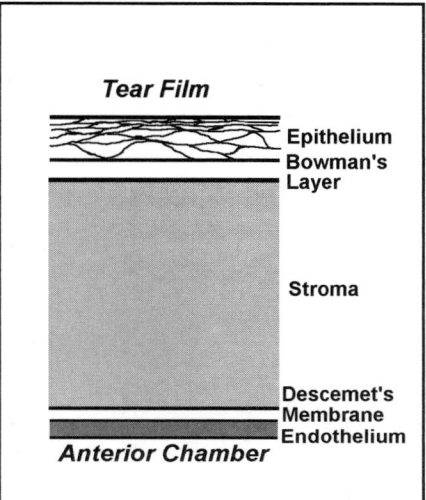

keratin layer is lacking in the eye. Most of the corneal thickness is provided by the *stroma*. Cells known as *keratocytes* are packed tightly with collagen and other structural proteins in a manner which allows it to be transparent. The front or anterior part of the stroma is known as *Bowman's layer*. Near the posterior aspect of the cornea is *Descemet's membrane*. The single layer of cells known collectively as the *endothelium* actually secretes the collagen which forms Descemet's membrane.

Physiology: The cornea is a unique tissue which must perform a number of functions. First and foremost, it is a watertight *barrier* which keeps the contents of the globe in their appropriate places. While it must keep out toxic chemicals, harmful bacteria, and wayward mosquitos, it must allow light to pass through. It must be *transparent*. Nowhere else in the human body must a tissue be transparent and mother nature has taken great steps to preserve this state. Fluid accumulation within the cornea greatly reduces its transparency so its cells are constantly working to keep it in a state of relative dehydration. In addition, nutrients and oxygen are provided by the tear film which covers the cornea and by the aqueous humor which circulates behind it. This allows the cornea to survive without blood vessels which would compromise its transparency.

If the oxygen supply to the cornea is interrupted, its health may be threatened. As you will see when we review contact lenses, steps must be taken to preserve adequate oxygen delivery.

THE IRIS AND THE PUPIL

Those beautiful blue eyes. Those mysterious brown eyes. It is the pigmentation of the iris which gives the eye its color. In addition, there are muscle layers in the iris which allow it to constrict and dilate.

When you look in the mirror, the pupil is the black circle in the very centre of the eye. In fact, the pupil is nothing more than the hole which is circumscribed by the iris.

THE CRYSTALLINE LENS

Anatomy: Behind the iris lies the crystalline lens. Also a transparent structure, it consists of a capsule, cells, and fibres. It is often referred to as simply the lens, but in order to avoid confusion with a camera lens, an intraocular lens, and a contact lens we will refer to it by its full name.

Physiology: In order to transmit light, the lens, like the cornea, must be transparent or nearly so. As we get older, the crystalline lens becomes larger and may become cloudy. An opacification in the crystalline lens is called a *cataract*. What is special about the crystalline lens is its ability to change

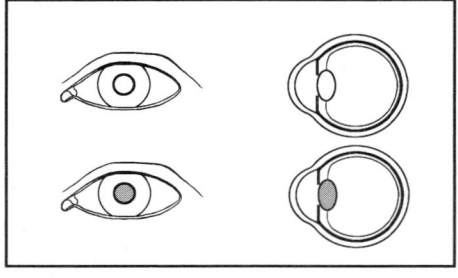

shape, depending on the activity of the muscles which attach to it. As we will see, this property allows the crystalline lens to assist in the focusing of light.

THE RETINA

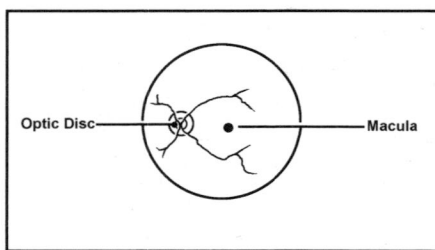

Anatomy: The retina is a complex 10-layered neurological tissue which lines the inside of the eye. It consists of photosensitive light receptors, nerves cells, nerve fibres, blood vessels, and a special group of cells known as the retinal pigment epithelium. At the back pole of the eye is a region known as the *macula*. It is this specialized area that is responsible for the fine central visual acuity which is so important for driving and reading.

Physiology: There are two kinds of photoreceptor cells in the retina, *rods* and *cones*. There are three kinds of cones, each of which contains a unique pigment which responds to a specific wavelength of light. The cones provide color vision and fine visual discrimination, and are concentrated in the macula. The rods, in a complementary fashion, contribute mainly to night vision, perception of movement, and peripheral vision.

When light reaches the retina, it is absorbed by one of these pigments and a chemical reaction ensues. A cascade of events follows which ultimately results in a nerve impulse being sent toward the brain through the optic nerve. When your brain interprets these impulses, originating from rods and cones scattered throughout the retina, you "see".

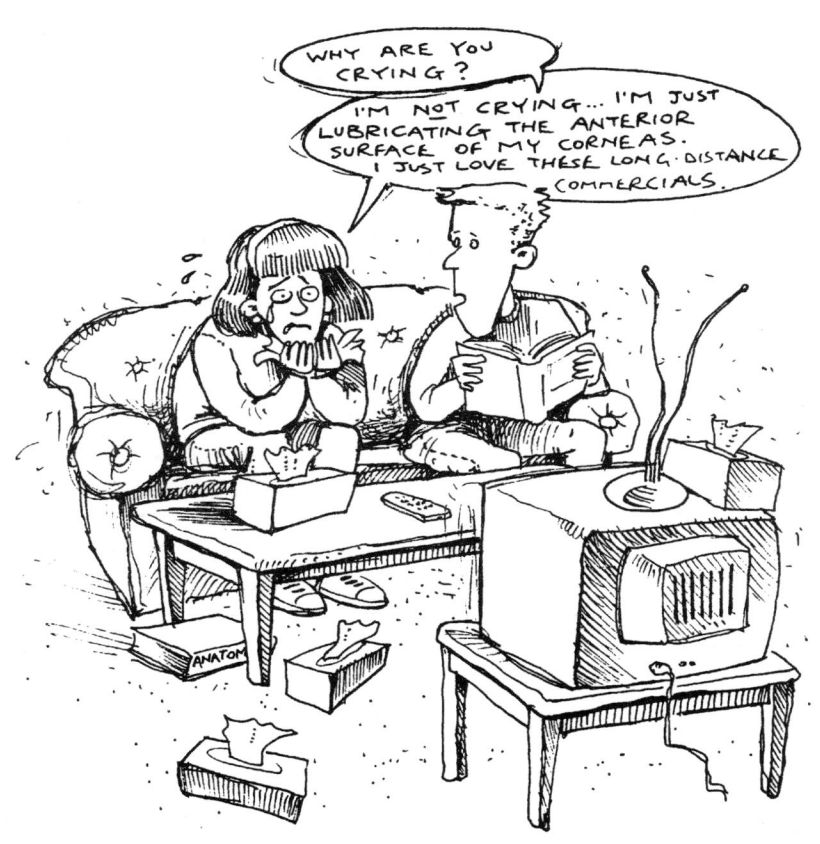

THE TEAR FILM

Anatomy: We only remember them when chopping onions, watching sad movies, or crying over spilled milk, but it is important that we do not forget about our tears. The three layers, from front to back, are the oily *lipid* layer, the watery *aqueous* layer, and the, well, mucousy *mucous* layer which lies right on the surface of the cornea.

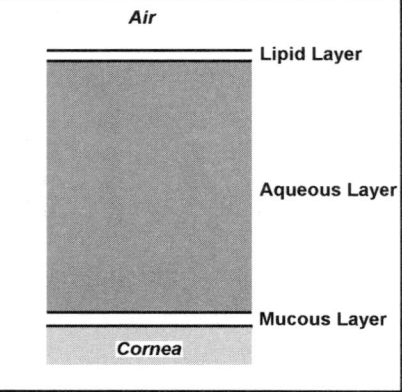

Physiology: The tear film serves many roles including protection, antisepsis, nutrition, and preservation of a smooth optical surface. Although we take our tears for granted, any deficiencies or dysfunction can have devastating consequences to the eye.

Focus

When last we saw you, you had thrown your camera to the ground. You were standing in front of a shiny red apple with your eyes open in anticipation. The red light which had reflected off the apple was moving pretty quickly (at the speed of light, in fact) toward your eyes. We now pick up the action as the light rays go through the cornea, the pupil, and the lens, before ending their stellar journey at retinal impact. If the light rays converge properly and focus on the retina, a clear image is formed.

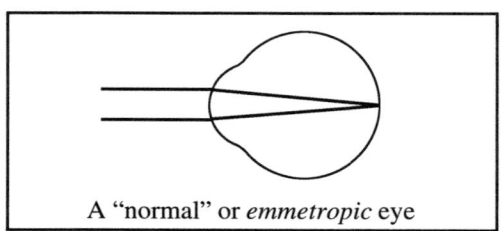

A "normal" or *emmetropic* eye

If, however, light does not focus properly on the retina, then the image we see is not clear. If this happens, a *refractive error* exists. For instance, light may be focussed in front of the retina.

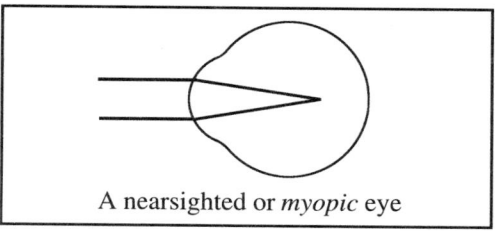

A nearsighted or *myopic* eye

Conversely, light may be focussed behind the retina.

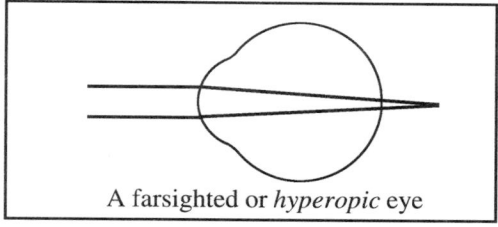

A farsighted or *hyperopic* eye

What determines where the light rays are focussed? In general, it depends on two factors. The first is the *refractive power* of the eye. When parallel light rays hit the cornea, they are bent or redirected, and start converging. When these bent light rays hit the lens, they are bent some more. If the cornea and lens bend the light rays by the just the right amount, they end up being focussed at exactly the right place, on the retina. If, for example, the cornea bends the light too much, because its refracting power is too *strong,* the light rays will focus in front of the retina causing nearsightedness. If the refracting power is too *weak,* the light will focus behind the retina resulting in farsightedness.

When we say the refracting power is too strong or too weak, these are relative terms. The second important factor is the length of the eyeball or *axial length.* If the eye has a "normal" or average refractive power, but the eye is longer than average, the light will end up being focussed in front of the retina. Conversely, a shorter globe combined with a normal refractive power will cause farsightedness.

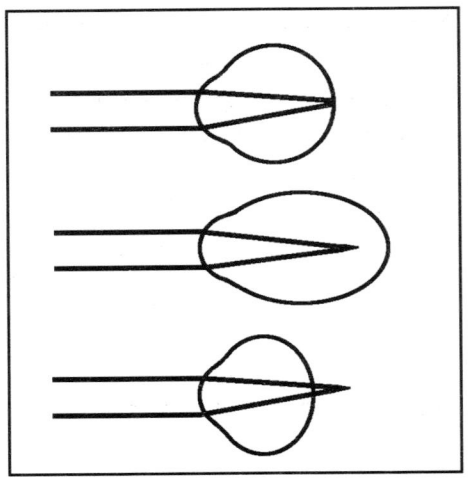

As you can see, it is the combination of refractive power and axial length which determines if you are nearsighted or farsighted.

NEARSIGHTEDNESS (MYOPIA)

There is a great deal of confusion over the subject. Quite simply, if you can see near objects well, but have trouble at a distance, you are nearsighted. Either your eyeball is too long or your refractive power is too strong or there is a combination of the two. Regardless of the cause, parallel light rays from a distant object are being focussed in front of the retina. The more myopic the eye, the farther the focus is from the retina and the more blurry the vision.

FARSIGHTEDNESS (HYPEROPIA)

If you have more trouble seeing near than far, then you are probably farsighted. Either the eyeball is too short or the refractive power is too weak. Parallel light rays from a distant object would focus behind the retina causing a blurred image. And as we shall soon see, divergent light from a near object would focus even farther behind the retina causing even more blurriness. (Hyperopia should not be confused with presbyopia which will be discussed later in this chapter).

ASTIGMATISM

If you examine a normal cornea, you will see that it is a spherical dome like a slice of a basketball or an orange.

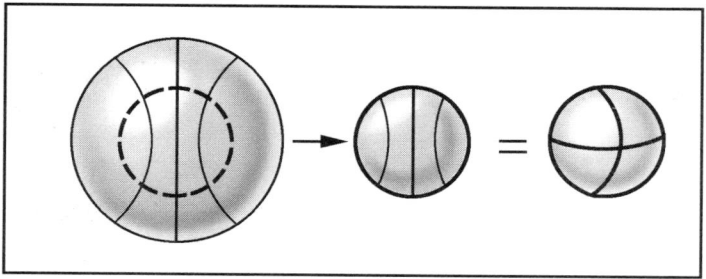

If you examine an eye with *regular* astigmatism, you will notice that it is more like a slice of a football or an egg.

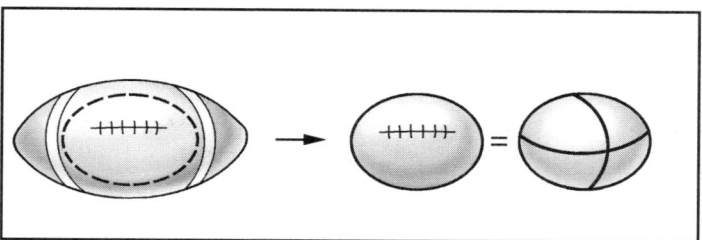

As you can see, its surface is curved more in one direction than in the other. The power, therefore, is stronger at one corneal meridian than in the other. This results in the image not being properly focussed on the retina.

Instead of creating a sharp point of an image, a blur circle is created. The greater the amount of astigmatism, the more unclear the image.

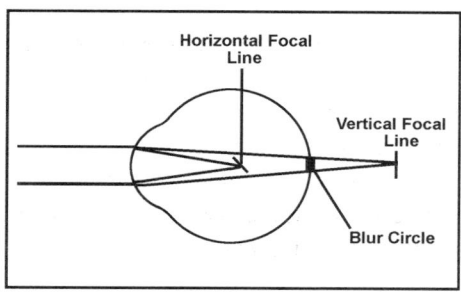

FROM NEAR TO ETERNITY

In our examples, we have been referring to parallel light rays. When you look at a far away object, its light rays are virtually parallel when they reach your eye. If however, you hold an apple in your hand, this assumption is not correct. The light rays from the apple are in fact diverging as they reach your eye. So in the eyes' resting state, the light rays would not be bent enough to focus on the retina. They would reach a focus behind the retina. The apple would be blurry.

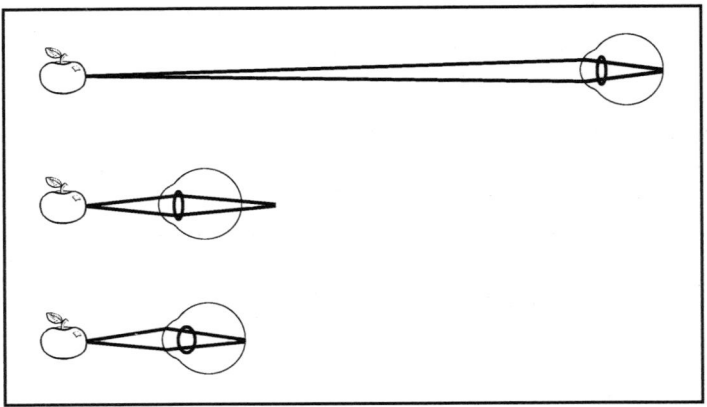

Because the light rays would be focussed behind the retina, you need to increase the refracting power of the eye to focus the light on the retina. This is where your crystalline lens comes into play. As you remember, the eye has the ability to change the shape of the crystalline lens. It is this ability which allows you to focus on near objects. When you look at a near object, the muscles inside your eye contract, making the crystalline lens more spherical. This is known as *accommodation*. It increases the refractive power of your eye thereby focussing the light rays from a near object onto your retina. You can see the apple in your hand.

PRESBYOPIA

Around the age of forty or forty-five, people who have never worn glasses before in their lives may start to behave strangely. They squint at their watches, they hold books at arms length, and they have trouble seeing that apple in their hands. And they complain that their arms are too short. And after they have been checked by their psychiatrists, as a last resort they go to see their eye doctor. Here's what is happening. The crystalline lens is becoming older, stiffer, and less able to do the things it used to do. It can no longer supply the eye with the additional refractive power that it needs to see things up close.

This is a normal, predictable aging phenomenon known as *presbyopia*. At the age of five, you could have impressed your kindergarten classmates with your ability to focus on a crayon at 2 inches. You could have held your first driver's license at 3 inches and still seen the acne on the photograph. However as inevitable as death and taxes, your crystalline lenses desert you just in time for your mid-life crisis.

If you were fortunate enough to be myopic all of your life, your years of frustration are finally rewarded. You have near sight. Taking off your glasses makes it unnecessary for you to have added refractive power to help with near vision. You have a set of built in reading glasses.

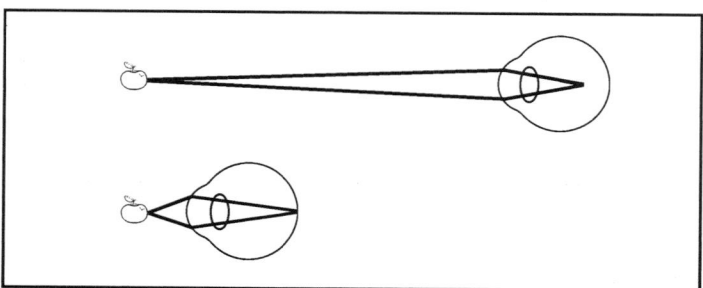

Depending on your degree of myopia, you may be the only one at the party who can read the menu without glasses.

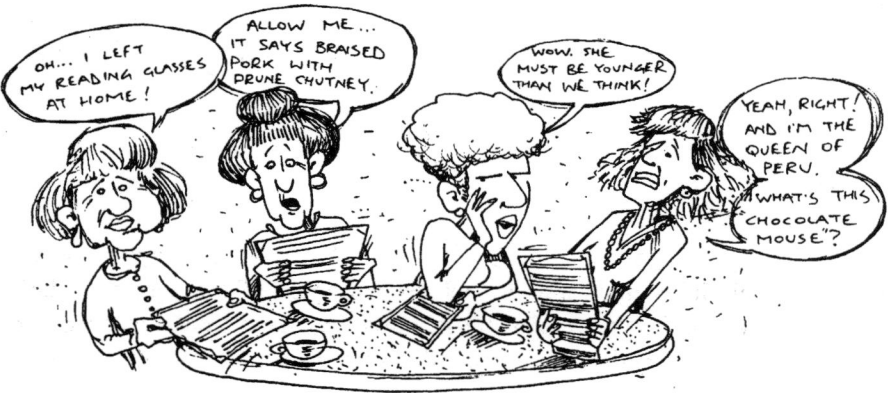

2

PUTTING NUMBERS
TO PICTURES

POWER

In order to try and solve the problems of nearsightedness and farsightedness, we need to be as accurate as possible. To quantify the power of any lens, we use the *Diopter*. One Diopter, or 1 D as it is commonly written, is defined as the power of a lens which can bring parallel light rays to a focus one meter away from the lens. A lens which is twice as strong, a 2 D lens, focusses the same light rays at half a meter.

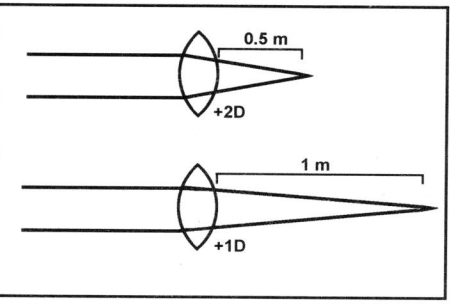

The cornea is a very powerful refractive surface. On average, it's power is approximately 42 D. The lens of the eye also acts as a refractive surface.

Combined, the cornea and lens act as an extremely powerful refracting surface of nearly 60 D. Parallel light rays are focussed approximately 22 millimetres (mm) or 7/8 of an inch from the front of the eye. By strange coincidence or design, this is usually the position of the retina.

In addition to its numerical value, each lens also has a sign. By convention, a *plus* (+) lens refers to a lens which causes light to converge. This is the kind of lens worn by hyperopes. The cornea and crystalline lens of the eye also act as plus lenses. A *minus* (-) lens causes light to diverge and is used to help nearsighted individuals. A *plano* (pl) lens has zero power and is just like a piece of plastic or glass.

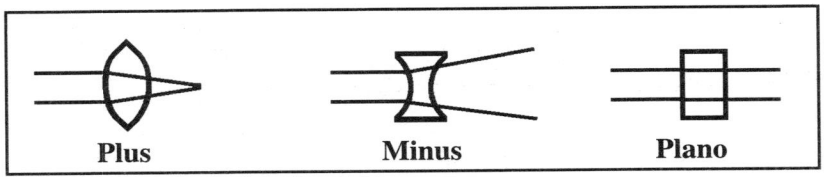

In a related manner, the Diopter can be used to quantify the refractive error of an eye. For example, a 3 D hyperope refers to a farsighted eye which requires a +3 D lens to focus the light on the retina. Conversely, a -3 lens is what a 3 Diopter myope wears to correct his or her nearsightedness.

WHAT IS 20/20?

There is a reason many health care professionals have selected 2020 as the last four digits in their telephone numbers. It has come to represent the gold standard. Perfect vision. And undoubtedly dialling 1-U2CANC2020 is a little more confidence inspiring than 1-BLINDASBAT.   Still, in our search for 20/20, we must go one step further. We must understand it.

You've heard the numbers. 20/20. 20/40. 20/200. What do they have in common? The first number in all of these fractions, the *numerator,* is 20. This refers to the testing distance, which is usually 20 feet. Most often, then, the visual acuity measurement will take the form of 20/x. Forget about the numerator. The important part of the fraction is the *denominator,* x, which is recorded from the eye chart.

If you have normal vision, you can see 20/20. This means that you can see the line labelled as "20" on the eye chart. If you can only see the fourth line from the bottom, the "40" line, then your vision is 20/40. The numbers on this line are so big, that a normal person can identify these letters at 40 feet. 20/200 vision means that in order to see what your normal friend can see from 200 feet away, you must walk up to 20 feet away.

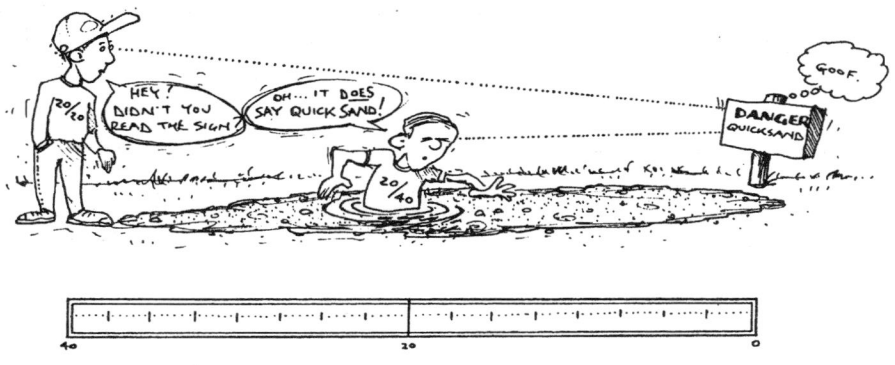

Therefore, 20/20 vision is better than 20/40 vision, which is itself better than 20/200.

You may hear the numbers 6/6 being thrown around. Or 6/15. Do not be alarmed. It's just that while we're still talking about feet, the metric system has become the international standard. In other countries, and increasingly in the United States, the numbers 6/6 are replacing 20/20. Meters are replacing feet. 6 meters is approximately 20 feet. Don't be alarmed. It doesn't change anything. It is the fraction which is important. 6/6 means the same thing as 20/20. 6/12 is 20/40 and so on. In fact, in some countries, the convention is to use decimals to express the visual acuity. For example, 20/20 is 1.0, and 20/40 is 0.5. However, for the sake of tradition, not to mention the title of this book, we will continue to talk about feet.

BEYOND **20/20**

When we assess the vision at 20 feet, we are referring to distance vision. There are ways to measure and record *near vision*. One of the most common ways is the use of a near card, which is a small version of an eye chart to be held at a specified distance.

When anyone's eyes are examined, visual acuity measurements are an essential component. As already mentioned, both *near* and *distance* vision are usually recorded. If glasses or contact lenses are not worn, the documented vision is *uncorrected*. Conversely, *corrected* vision refers to the visual acuity obtained with you, the patient, wearing your glasses or contact lenses. You may recall visiting your eye doctor and having them flip several lenses in front of your eyes. They asked you which lenses made things better and which ones made things worse. After what seemed like hours of pushing and prodding, some numbers were scribbled down. With this prescription, what you see is your *best-corrected* vision.

If the patient's vision is so poor that he or she cannot read the top letter on the eye chart, we then check if they can count fingers (CF), detect hand motion (HM), or perceive/localize light (LP).

THE PINHOLE

After years of procrastination, you finally decided to get your eyes checked. The doctor you selected came highly recommended by the same friends who suggested *Il Postino*. You found her office filled with all of these state of the art gadgets and a bunch of impressive certificates which spelled out her middle name in full. The examination was going well until this doctor pulled out a high tech piece of plastic with a high tech pinhole in it. She held it up to your eye and had the audacity to ask you if it cleared things up a little. And it did.

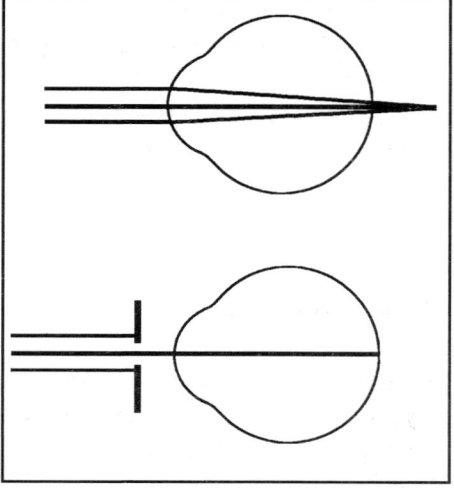

The pinhole acts to compensate for your refractive error. Any improvement in visual acuity when looking through a pinhole can be attributed to nearsightedness, farsightedness, or astigmatism. It is not quite as accurate as more advanced techniques, but it is a useful tool. The pinhole, quite simply, gives an indication of *potential* vision.

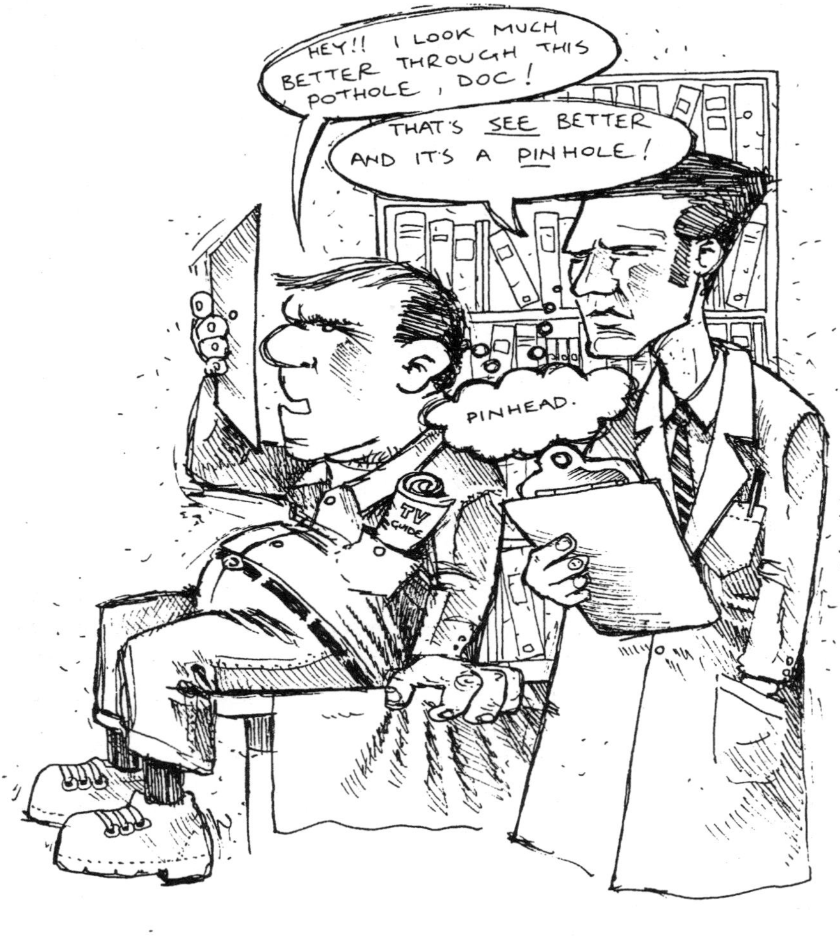

VISION REQUIREMENTS

In order to prevent visually impaired people from joining their psychologically stunted, manner deficient, and directionally challenged colleagues on the roads, certain visual requirements must be met. The actual criteria vary from location to location, so it is advisable to check the specifics with your local authorities. In general, however, there is a *visual acuity* standard and a *visual field* standard.

The visual acuity standard refers to a minimum distance acuity. Depending on the type of license, there may be specified required vision in each eye or simply a minimum visual acuity with both eyes open. 20/40 is often used as the cutoff.

Your visual field refers to the amount of peripheral vision you have. People who have glaucoma, for example, may have 20/20 vision, however their side vision may be reduced to a 30 degree field. Imagine trying to drive a car with such tunnel vision.

LEGAL BLINDNESS

I remember a person running into my office crying, "I'm going blind, Doc! I'm going blind!". As I stood across the room from him, he proceeded to compliment me on the design etched on my tie-clip. Although it is quite understandable to be concerned by any drop in vision, no matter how small, the term blind should be reserved for certain specific situations. Legal blindness is defined as a best-corrected vision of 20/200 or less, or a visual field of less than 10%.

3

To See or Not To See

So you can't see. You're nearsighted, farsighted, or astigmatic. What are the options

The Options

I. Do nothing

II. Use the natural abilities of your eyes
    A. Squinting
    B. Accommodation

III. Put something in front of your eyes (Chapter 3)
    A. Pinhole
    B. Glasses
    C. Contact lenses

continued....

IV. Have surgery

    A. Change the refractive surface of the cornea

        1. Conventional surgery

            a. Use linear radial cuts which allows the cornea to assume a flatter shape (RK - Chapter 7)

            b. Use arcuate cuts which allows the cornea to assume a more spherical shape (AK - Chapter 9)

            c. Use hexagonal cuts which allows the cornea to assume a steeper shape (HK - Chapter 10)

            d. Use a blade to remove corneal tissue, thereby flattening it (ALK - Chapter 6)

            e. Use a blade to weaken the cornea, thereby allowing it to bulge and steepening it (ALK - Chapter 10)

        2. Laser surgery

            a. Use laser to remove corneal tissue, thereby flattening or steepening it (PRK - Chapter 5, LASIK - Chapter 6)

            b. Use laser to change the shape of the cornea thermally (Holmium:YAG LTK - Chapter 10)

        3. Investigational surgery

            a. Implant material into the cornea to change its shape (ICRS - Chapter 11)

    B. Change the refractive power inside the eye

        1. Replace the crystalline lens with an intraocular lens implant (Cataract extraction, refractive lensectomy Chapter 8)

        2. Implant an intraocular lens without removing the crystalline lens (Phakic IOL, Intraocular contact lens Chapter 11)

DO NOTHING

So you see 20/60. You remember somebody giving you a prescription 5 years ago. You recall selecting some fancy frames, deciding on just the right tint, and giving the optician a sizeable cheque. And where are these glasses now? They are gathering dust on a shelf beside your Rubik's cube. Is this a problem? Should you be wearing glasses?

The short answer is that it is up to you. The reason someone prescribed glasses for you was that they thought it would improve your vision. But if you don't drive a car, and if you don't have any trouble watching television or doing any of the things that you like to do, then that's fine. With a few exceptions, *you're not going to harm your eyes by not wearing glasses*. And you're not going to improve your eyes by wearing glasses. All glasses do is bend the light to focus it on the retina. As soon as you take off your glasses, your eyes are the same as they were before. Yes, doing nothing can be a reasonable option. In our 'Should I buy a car?' analogy, there is nothing wrong with walking.

There are a couple of important exceptions. Young children who wear glasses need them in order to ensure that their visual system develops properly. If the correct glasses aren't worn, a lazy or *amblyopic* eye can mean permanent visual loss. Also, *protective* glasses should be worn in certain circumstances, not to improve the vision, but to prevent visual loss. This is especially important for people with only one good eye.

SQUINTING

You don't need a book to tell you that squinting can make things clearer. What you are doing, in fact, is narrowing your eyelid fissure, thereby simulating a pinhole. As we described earlier, looking through a pinhole improves your vision when the visual loss is due to a refractive error. So if you're nearsighted and you have trouble seeing a road sign, squinting brings the words into focus. You don't have to buy a car when you can hop in a cab whenever you want.

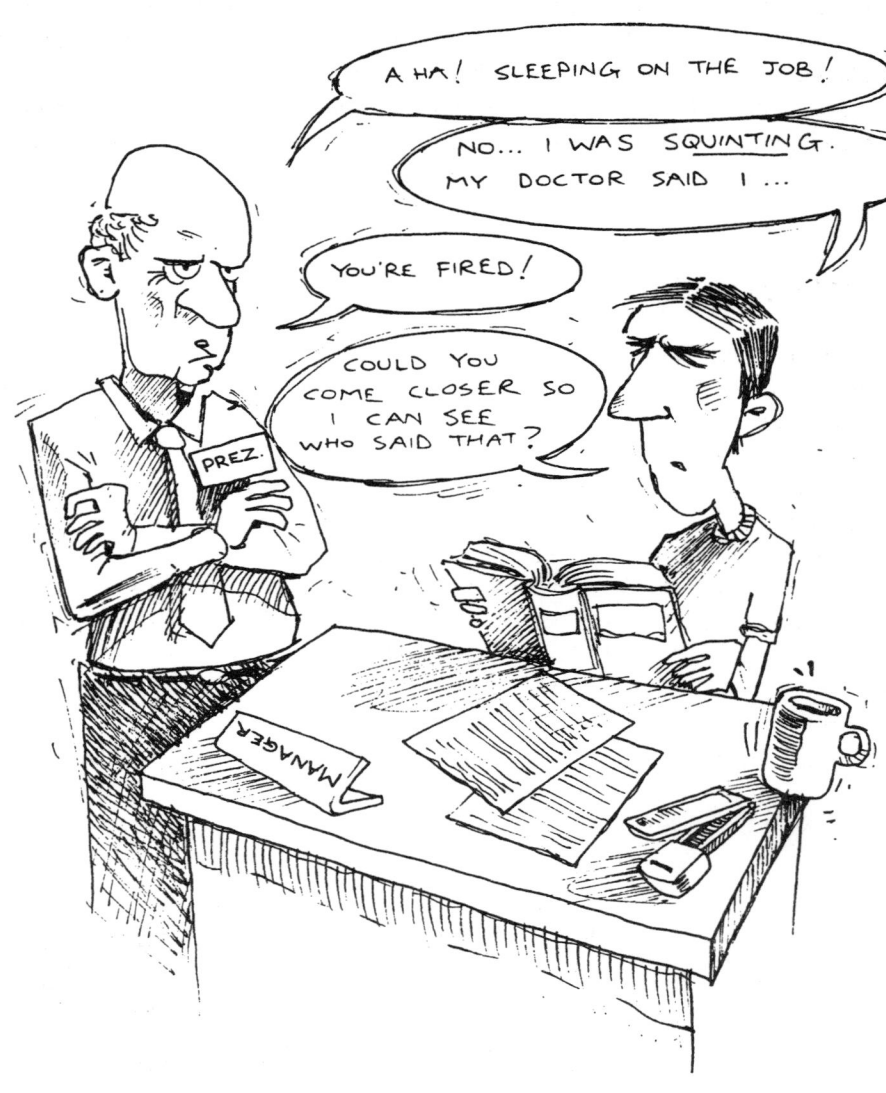

PINHOLES

Instead of using your eyelids to make a pinhole, why not just hold a pinhole up against your eye? You may have seen them advertised on television, glasses with little pinholes in each lens. As you now know, there is nothing magical about these glasses. It is just the pinhole effect which acts to improve the vision. It's like taking the bus. It gets you where you want to go, but it may not be the most fashionable way to travel.

ACCOMMODATION

As you recall, when you want to read something up close, the shape of your crystalline lens changes. This gives your eye the extra power it needs to focus light from a near object onto your retina. If you are farsighted, you can also take advantage of this mechanism to counteract your refractive error. A 2 Diopter hyperope, who has trouble seeing distant objects, can use his or her accommodation to supply the missing 2 D of power. The distant image becomes clear. In order to see well up close, this same person needs to use an *additional* amount of accommodative power, over and above the 2 D. Regardless, accommodation can result is clear vision, without the use of glasses or contacts.

At what cost? You can borrow your friend's car, but if you do it too often or for too long, you may put a strain on the relationship. Similarly, if the degree

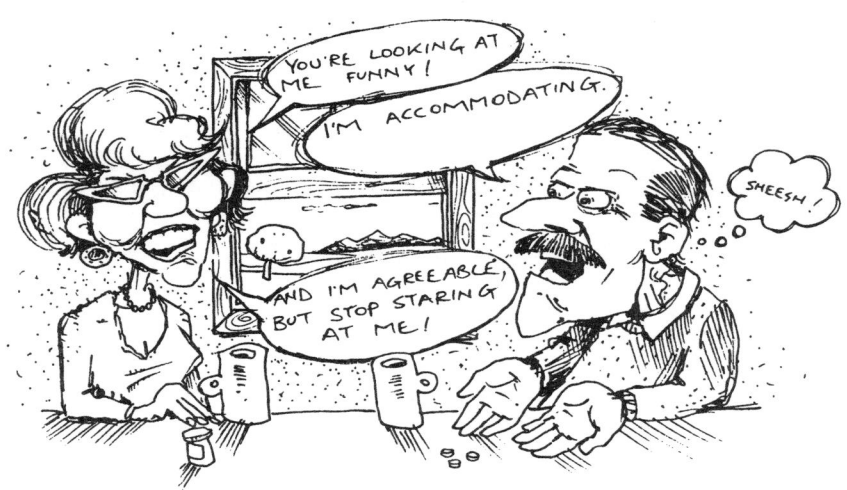

of hyperopia is too great, eyestrain symptoms can result. Headaches can develop or the eyes may become fatigued after short periods of reading. Furthermore, as the hyperope gets older, the *accommodative reserve* diminishes, and this built in mechanism may no longer be adequate. Therefore, although accommodation is a useful tool for hyperopes, it is not necessarily an ideal or permanent solution.

GLASSES

So your feet are tired. You can't stand taking the bus and your former friend refuses to lend you her wheels. It's time to buy a car. It's time to talk about glasses.

How they work

In general, glasses act to focus light on the retina. The type of lens in the glasses depends on the refractive error.

Hyperopic correction: As mentioned earlier, the problem here is that the light is focussed behind the retina.

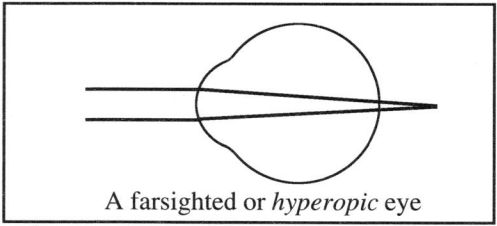

A farsighted or *hyperopic* eye

In order to focus the light on the retina, we can put a lens in front of the eye. This lens, must act to converge light. It is, by definition, a plus (+) lens.

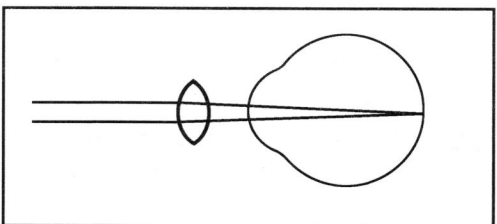

Myopic correction: A myopic eye, conversely, has light rays from a distant object focusing in front of the retina.

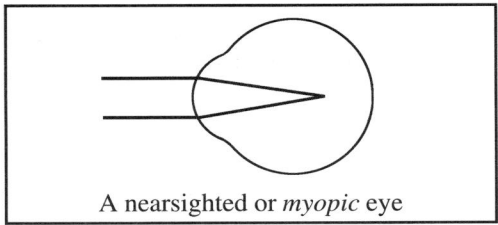

A nearsighted or *myopic* eye

It requires a lens which diverges light rays, or a minus (-) lens.

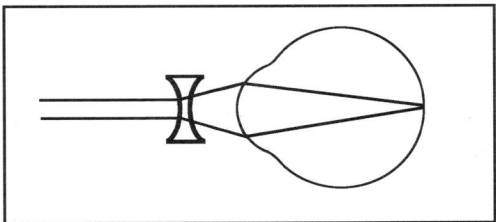

Astigmatic correction: An astigmatic eye is a little more complicated. As you recall, the cornea of the astigmatic eye is analogous to a slice off a football. Let's take this football and put it on it's side. A football, as you know, does not like to stand up vertically. *As a rule*, it prefers to lie on its side.

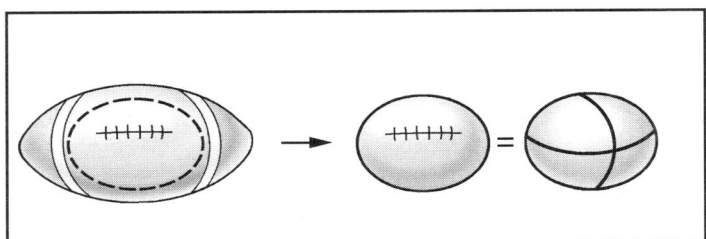

This cornea has two power *meridians*. In the following example, one meridian focusses light behind the retina. The other meridian is more curved, however, and is a stronger refracting surface. So it focusses light in front of the retina.

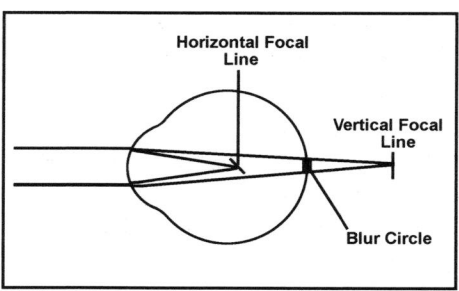

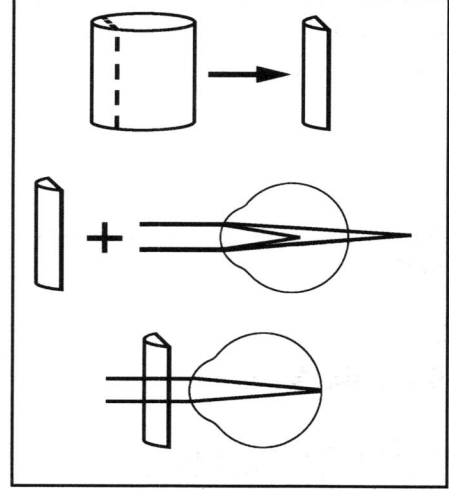

So instead of creating a focal point on the retina, two focal lines are created. The goal of prescribing glasses is to push these two lines together, creating a single point of focus on the retina. And this is done using a *cylindrical lens* (or *cylinder* for short).

A cylinder is a type of lens which has power in one meridian but not in the other.

A cylinder can be described by its *power* and by its *axis*. Let's go back to our football which, as a rule, tends to lie on its side. If we put a cylinder of the appropriate power in the appropriate axis, in front of this eye, the two focal lines will move together to form a single focal point. When using plus cylinder notation, the axis of the correcting cylinder in this situation is vertical or at 90 degrees. This is known as *with-the-rule* astigmatism.

If the football is standing on its end, the more powerful meridian is now horizontal. This is *against-the-rule* astigmatism and the axis of the plus correcting cylinder is 180 degrees.

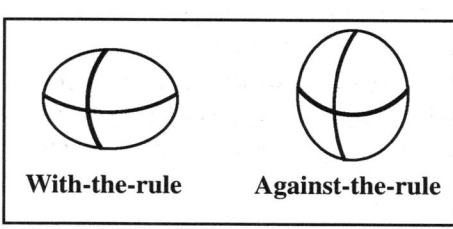

With-the-rule   **Against-the-rule**

The important thing to realize about astigmatism is that there are two components involved. The power of the correcting cylinder and its axis of orientation.

All of this refers to regular astigmatism. *Irregular* astigmatism, is more of a problem. It is variable, uncorrectable by glasses or soft-contact lenses, and may be responsible for the loss of best-corrected visual acuity following refractive surgery.

Presbyopic correction: In order to compensate for a presbyope's insufficient accommodative ability, additional *plus* power must be added to the distance correction. The amount of power to be added depends on the patient's age, accommodative reserve, and preferred reading distance.

The Prescription

See if you can find an old prescription from your eye doctor. Now see if you can read it. Chances are, it looks something like this:

OD -2.50
OS   -3.50 + 2.00 X 90

OD is short for *oculus dexter* and means *right eye.*
OS is short for *oculus sinister* and means *left eye.*
OU is short for *oculi uterque* and means *both eyes.*

The numbers fit the following equation:

Sphere +/- Cylinder Power X Cylinder Axis
(The units of the sphere and cylinder are
in Diopters. The axis is in degrees.)

The sphere corrects the nearsightedness or farsightedness and the cylinder corrects the astigmatism. If there is no cylinder, only the sphere is recorded. This means that there is no astigmatism. In the example above, we know that the right eye has 2.50 D of myopia, because the sign is negative. We also know that the right eye has no astigmatism, because no correcting cylinder was prescribed.

The left eye has 3.50 D of myopia but also exhibits astigmatism. The correcting cylinder is 2.00 D positioned with its axis at 90 degrees.

In the situation where there is only astigmatism and no correcting sphere is required, the abbreviation pl is used to signify plano, or just a powerless piece of plastic.

$$\text{eg: pl + 1.50 X 180}$$

If your prescription is for bifocals, your doctor will have written something like:

$$\textbf{Add} = +2.00$$

The *add* refers to the additional 2 D of power that you require for reading vision.

One final word. It is important to note that your prescription can be written in two different forms:

$$-2.50 + 1.00 \text{ X } 90$$

is actually exactly the same prescription as

$$-1.50 - 1.00 \text{ X } 180$$

The only difference is that one is written in *plus* cylinder form and one is written in *minus* cylinder form. They are interchangeable and if you gave both prescriptions to your optician, you would get the same lens. It is not important to know how to convert from one to the other. It is good to be aware, however, that if two doctors give you two prescriptions which look nothing like each other, it doesn't necessarily mean that one of them is out to lunch.

So you have trouble seeing. You've had enough of squinting, accommodating, and looking through nerdy pinhole glasses. You are interested in getting some real glasses and you want to know the pluses and minuses. That is, uh, the pros and cons.

Pros

Safety: The medical world operates under the principle, 'First, do no harm'. In real terms, whenever someone needs treatment for a medical condition, noninvasive techniques are preferred over more risky invasive measures. If someone's heart is failing, medicine is used before open heart surgery is advised.

The least invasive treatment of a refractive error is the prescription of glasses. Resting on your nose and ears, they offer no threat to your eyes. In fact, polycarbonate lenses actually protect the eyes. More important is what glasses do not do. They do not sit on your corneas, nor do they cut, shape, or otherwise affect your eyes themselves. All glasses do is bend the light, allowing an image to focus on the retina. If you want to improve your vision with minimal risk, glasses are the Volvos of the ophthalmic world.

Simplicity: You can see your eye doctor in the morning and be reading a lunchtime menu. The prescription and construction of the lenses are easy. And unlike contact lenses, learning how to wear glasses is not an issue. In fact, probably the most difficult step in the whole process is choosing the perfect frame.

Intermittence: If you have a very small refractive error, you may feel that your vision is good enough for most activities. Perhaps you only have trouble seeing the fine print in your biology class, where you have to sit in the back row to avoid being picked on by your myopic professor. You pull out your glasses at the beginning of the class and stow them away at the end. Glasses are great for intermittent use.

Bifocals: If you are at the age where you need additional power for near vision, bifocals are a great solution. Here you have two lenses in one. When you want to read, you look through the bottom part of the glasses. When you want to see far away, you look through the top. Although there can be some difficulty adjusting to them for the first time, bifocals are a good way (but not the only way) of dealing with presbyopia.

Cons

Cosmetic: Some people don't like the way they look in glasses. Just like some people don't like the way they look in stripes. Or in Volvos. It's a matter of personal preference.

Sports: When was the last time you saw a professional hockey player wearing glasses? With all those fists in their face, their entire salary would be spent on new glasses, and they wouldn't be able to afford new teeth. Although some athletes can get away with glasses, there is a trend toward the other alternatives.

Visual changes: Depending on the power and nature of your prescription, you may encounter a variety of visual phenomena when you wear your glasses. In general, the greater the prescription, the more pronounced the effect. Some people are quite immune to these changes while others are more sensitive.

> ***Minification/Magnification:*** If you are nearsighted try the following experiment. Look at an object without your glasses. Now look at the same object with your glasses on. Do you notice any difference in the size? Myopes, as a rule, observe that objects appear smaller with their glasses on. Hyperopes, conversely, appreciate an apparent magnification of the object. The degree of minification/magnification corresponds with the degree of myopia/hyperopia. If both eyes have a similar refractive error, then this effect may not cause much of a problem. If, however, the two eyes are quite different, then difficulties may arise.
>
> ***Anisometropia*** is defined as a significant difference in the refractive error of the two eyes. While most people have eyes which are similar to each other, it is unusual to find eyes which are identical. So when we talk about anisometropia, we usually refer to a significant difference between the two eyes. Significant is defined to be around 2 D.
>
> If one eye has 1 D of myopia and the other has 2 D of myopia, there is a difference in the image size when wearing glasses. The more myopic eye will appreciate a smaller image. With a difference of 1 D, however, the size difference is insignificant. That is, the brain has the ability to fuse these two slightly different images into single binocular vision. At anything over 2 D of anisometropia, the difference becomes too great for the brain to resolve. Wearing glasses becomes a problem.
>
> ***Peripheral Vision***: Stare at a spot straight ahead. Keep looking

there. Now pull one hand behind you as if you were taking a tennis backswing. Slowly bring it forward until you can see it. Notice the position of your hand. It's pretty much beside you. If you do the same thing with the other hand, you will realize that you have pretty good peripheral vision. Even though you don't have eyes at the back of your head, you can still see about 180 degrees in front of you without moving your eyes. Unfortunately, glasses do not extend for the full half-circle. Therefore, although wearing glasses improves your straight ahead vision, your peripheral vision is largely uncompensated. This is even more pronounced if you keep your head still and move your eyes all the way to one side. You will find yourself looking *around* your glasses instead of through them.

Distortion: Let's examine an eye which is very farsighted. An example of this is someone who has had a cataract removed, but for whatever reason, has had no lens implant inserted. A high plus lens is required to improve the visual acuity. Wearing these glasses would cause the person to see a perfect square as a *pincushion*.

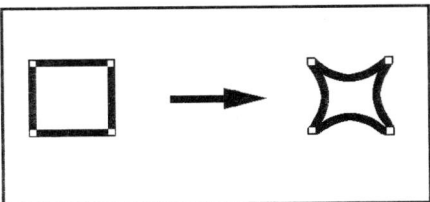

A very myopic individual who wears glasses will observe the opposite. This is known as *barrel* distortion.

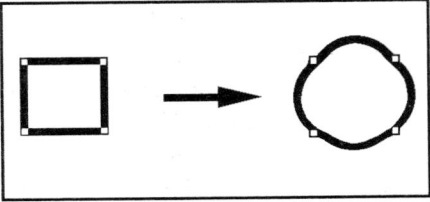

Bifocal problems: Image jump, image displacement, and a reduction of the peripheral visual field are not uncommonly associated with bifocal use.

CONTACT LENSES

How they work

Corrective lenses don't have to be restricted to glasses. They can be closer to the eye, as in contact lenses, or even inside the eye in the case of implants following cataract surgery. In the overall scheme of things, where we organize treatment from least invasive to most invasive, contact lenses are slightly more invasive than glasses. The reason is quite simple. When we put a contact lens against the eye, there is now an interface between the lens itself and the cornea. Because of this interface, problems can potentially develop.

Choices

There are a number of different kinds of contact lenses:

Polymethyl methacrylate (PMMA)

These lenses are rarely used these days, having largely been replaced by RGP lenses.

Rigid Gas Permeable (RGP)

As their name suggests, these lenses allow oxygen to be transferred across the contact lens to the cornea. In addition, because of the fact that they are rigid, these lenses have the special ability to compensate for corneal astigmatism. When placed on an astigmatic cornea, they change the refracting surface into a spherical one. Now, when light first reaches the eye, it hits a basketball, not a football. Therefore, RGP lenses have a unique role in the treatment of astigmatism.

Soft Contact Lenses (SCL)

In contrast to RGP lenses, soft contact lenses mold to the shape of the cornea. This means that whatever astigmatism was present in the cornea is not altered by the SCL. A football remains a football.

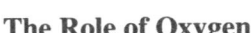

The Role of Oxygen

In order to preserve the health of the cornea, oxygen must be delivered to its cells. A rate-limiting step in the evolution of contact lenses has been its *oxygen transmissibility* which is defined as:

$$\frac{\text{Diffusion coefficient} \quad X \quad \text{Oxygen solubility}}{\text{Thickness of the lens}}$$

This means that the nature of the lens material correlates with the oxygen permeability. As technology is advancing, newer polymers are becoming available, which offer improved oxygen transmissibility. Furthermore, there is a trend toward thinner lenses which also means improved oxygen flow. These newer techniques and improved materials have revolutionized contact lenses in the last few years.

More Choices

Daily wear lenses, which used to be the standard lens of choice, are being challenged by *disposable* lenses. *Extended wear* lenses, with excellent oxygen transmissibility, allow periods of continued use without compromising the health of the cornea.

I Hate Bifocals

So you can't see the book in front of your face yet the thought of bifocals drives you crazy. Can contact lenses help treat presbyopia or should you make a reservation at the bifocal asylum? Here are your alternatives.

> **Option 1**: If you are slightly nearsighted and can see well up close without any correction, then you can take advantage of this fact. You can wear contact lenses for far away and pop them out when you need to see up close. Impractical for most people, but an option nonetheless.

> **Option 2**: You can wear contact lenses for distance vision and reading glasses over them when you need help up close.

Option 3: You can wear contact lenses of two different strengths. Your right eye. for example, can use a lens with the correct power for distance vision. Meanwhile, your left lens is strong enough to allow you to see near. This is called *monovision*. It takes a bit of getting used to, but the thinking is that you have two eyes. Why not put them both to work?

Option 4: Bifocal contact lenses. Some people love them, others hate them. *Translating* lenses act similarly to bifocal glasses. There are two distinct segments to look through, one for near and one for distance. *Simultaneous vision* lenses act by focusing two images on your retinas at the same time. It then becomes your job to pick which one you want to look at. The near image or the distant image. This can be a tricky proposition, however some people adapt very well. Keep watching, because every year, they get better and better.

Pros

Cosmetic: Contact lenses are life's red convertibles. They get you where you want to go in style. That is the main reason why contact lenses have become a multi-million dollar industry. Many people feel that they look better with contact lenses. Not only that, they see better. And so they feel better. An ancient proverb says that if you look better, see better, and feel better, then you might as well just do it.

Colored contacts: First it was hair color. Now this. Gone are the days when you are stuck with your baby blue eyes. If you are unhappy with what your parents gave you, it is no longer necessary to sue them for your pain and suffering. Now your eye doctor can override your genes. Simply insert a contact lens and voila, a brown-eyed girl.

Sports: They don't fog up, fall off (usually), or break when you get punched in the face during a hockey game. Sure, occasionally you will see an athlete on all fours, desperately searching the football field for an escaped lens. But by and large, people who are active in sports swear by contact lenses and wonder how they ever managed without them.

Astigmatism: As previously mentioned, contact lenses have a special ability to counteract astigmatism. The clarity of vision which a highly astigmatic person receives through contact lenses is unsurpassed. An extreme example of this is *keratoconus,* a disease of the cornea which results in high degrees of irregular astigmatism. Contact lenses are in fact the treatment of choice for this condition.

High myopia/hyperopia: The problems of image magnification/minification are most pronounced in individuals with a large refractive error. For example, if someone were to require a +12 D lens in their glasses, the image would be magnified about 25%. With the use of contact lenses, this can be reduced to about 7%, which is much easier to deal with.

Say that the right eye required the +12 D prescription but the left eye needed nothing. Imagine trying to walk around with a normal image in one eye and a much larger image in the other eye. Your poor brain would be unable to fuse the two images. Instead, if you wore a contact lens in your right eye, the size difference would be more manageable. Although this is an extreme example, the same approach applies with any significant degree of anisometropia. Wearing contact lenses will reduce the size discrepancy and improve the binocular vision.

Cons

The Learning Curve: It used to be that if you needed a good laugh, you found someone who had never gone windsurfing before in their lives and you gave them their first lesson. This has been replaced, as a comedic event, by watching someone experiment with contacts for the first time. For some reason, novices seem to believe that it is possible to get a lens on the cornea with the eyelids clenched tightly shut. Before you lens wearers snicker audibly, try and remember your first time. It isn't easy at the beginning. Just getting the lens in the right place is difficult. And if you do manage to succeed, it feels like there is something in your eye. (There is.) Then there are the cleaning and storage rituals. Fortunately, with some persistence and training, even most eye-shy people are able to wear contact lenses.

But not everybody. There are a number of people who just cannot deal with the thought of putting something in their eyes. It is quite understandable really. The blink reflex is a protective mechanism developed by the human body. It goes against natural reflexes to happily stick a finger in your eye.

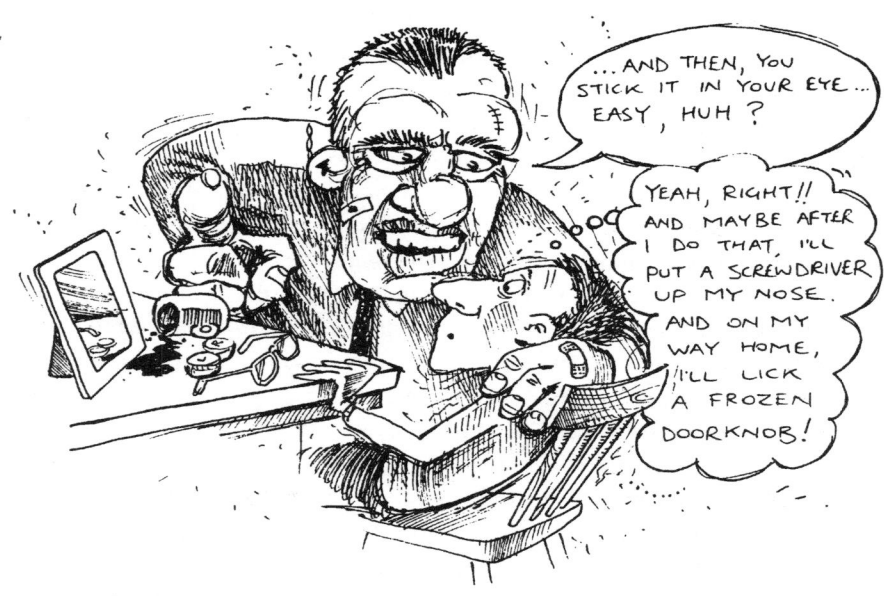

There is also a subset of people who have ocular conditions which prevent them from wearing contact lenses. Still another group becomes contact lens intolerant after having successfully worn contact lenses in the past. For a number of reasons, therefore, there are individuals who are either unable or unwilling to wear contact lenses.

Vision: As you know, RGP lenses have the ability to treat astigmatism. There are special soft contact lenses known as soft toric lenses, which also can be used to treat some types of astigmatism. Regular soft lenses, however, do not have the ability to counteract astigmatism. Yet these are the most common (and most inexpensive) type of contact lens. Say you have a small amount of astigmatism. Here the corrective cylinder was probably built into your glasses giving you crystal clear vision. Now if you move to regular soft contact lenses, this astigmatism is not corrected. Depending on the amount of astigmatism, the vision can be more blurry with your brand-new contacts than with your old glasses.

The Pre-Presbyopic Myope: _Pre-presbyopic_ means just before the age where reading glasses become necessary. So what we're talking about here is a person in their late thirties or early forties who is nearsighted. Typically, this

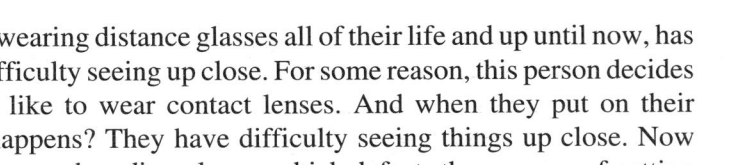

person has been wearing distance glasses all of their life and up until now, has never had any difficulty seeing up close. For some reason, this person decides that they would like to wear contact lenses. And when they put on their contacts, what happens? They have difficulty seeing things up close. Now they find that they need reading glasses which defeats the purpose of getting contact lenses in the first place. Rather than bore and confuse you with some impressive diagrams explaining why this happens, suffice it to say that if you are a pre-presbyopic myope, be aware of this potential problem.

Risks: We all know that convertibles are safe cars. Still, that doesn't mean you want to be driving in one if it rolls over. Although contact lenses are used safely by thousands around the world, problems can still occur and it is a good idea to be aware of them.

Oxygen problems: The health of the cornea is dependent on its receiving an adequate oxygen supply. Wearing a contact lens in itself can interfere somewhat with oxygen transmission. With the eyelid closed, the oxygen supply to the cornea is reduced even further. Therefore, unless the contact lens is sufficiently permeable to oxygen, wearing them for extended periods of time can jeopardize the health of the cornea. For this reason, it is generally inadvisable to sleep wearing your contact lenses.

Immune problems: When you get right down to it, the contact lens is nothing but a foreign object sitting in the eye. And sometimes, this is how the human body sees it. On occasion, the immune system can develop a reaction to the contact lens, to components of the cleaning/storage solutions, or to associated proteins. Contact lens intolerance can result.

Mechanical problems: With fingernails, contact lenses, and eye drops flying around the eye, it is not surprising to learn that the cornea can be threatened. Corneal abrasion, distortion, and stippling can occur with the use of contact lenses.

Infectious problems: You are surrounded by a jungle of microscopic organisms. Anytime you have a foreign object in proximity to the cornea, there is a chance an infection can develop. Bacteria, viruses, and amoeba have been known to attack the cornea with potentially devastating consequences.

Fortunately, it is a relatively rare occurrence. Still, every contact lens wearer should know that education, awareness, meticulous lens care, and regular visits to an eye care professional all play a vital role in maintaining the health of your eyes.

MEETING THE DOCTOR

Studies demonstrate that 70% of Americans believe that ophthalmologists are medical doctors, while 50% believe that optometrists are. Before you learn all about refractive eye surgery, it may be helpful to know a little bit about who is involved.

WHO'S WHO?

The Ophthalmologist

Ophthalmologists are physicians. Just like a cardiologist or an orthopedic surgeon, they are "doctors". Their typical training consists of a four year undergraduate degree, followed by a four year M.D. (Doctor of Medicine) or D.O. (Doctor of Osteopathy) degree. From there, they do a one year internship where they rotate through a combination of medicine, surgery, pediatrics, emergency medicine, and/or subspecialty training. In their tenth year of post-secondary education, they begin their ophthalmology program. This residency is another three or four years, where they begin by learning ocular anatomy, physiology, pathology, and pharmacology. In addition to examining and treating outpatients, performing refractions and contact lens fittings, their training includes laser and surgical procedures. When they graduate as fully-trained general ophthalmologists, many elect to enter the workforce. Others decide to pursue subspecialty training, spending one or more years narrowing their focus. Among the subspecialties are vitreoretinal surgery, neuro-ophthalmology, pediatric ophthalmology, anterior segment surgery, and refractive surgery. In total, a typical ophthalmologist may have been in training for thirteen or fourteen years after high school, and first ventures into the real world in their thirties.

After satisfactory completion of the residency program, an individual is considered to be a *Board Eligible* ophthalmologist. This means that they have fulfilled the training requirements of the American Board of Ophthalmology, are able to practice their craft, and that they are eligible to take the exams. The written examination is first, and if this is passed, they are offered the pleasure of taking the oral examination. If, after that, the paper inside the envelope says that they have passed, they are then considered *Board Certified* and have earned the privilege to call themselves "Diplomates of the American Board of Ophthalmology".

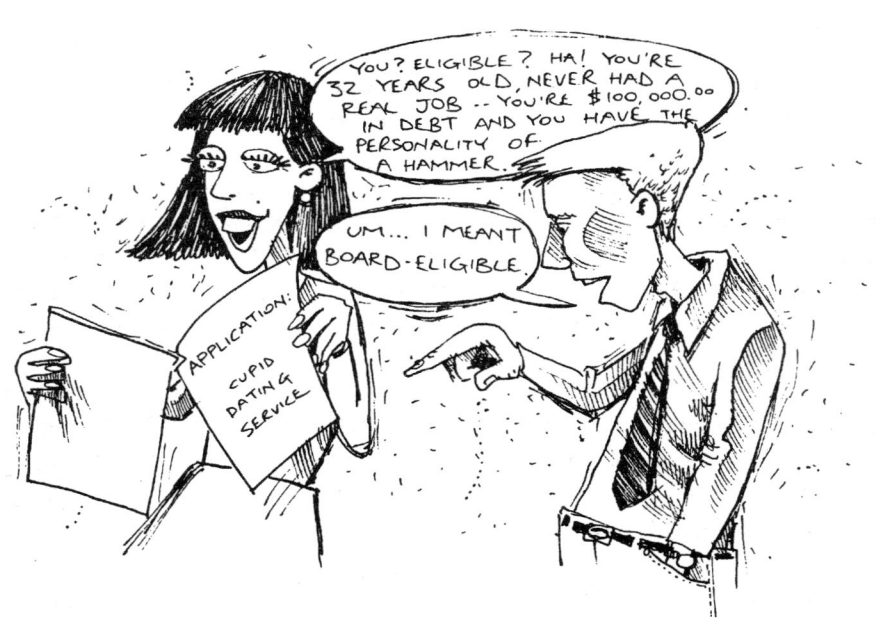

In Canada, the certifying board is called the Royal College of Physicians and Surgeons. Following satisfactory completion of a residency program, the exams must be taken. Again, there is a written and oral component. Those who pass are entitled to add a few letters after their name. F.R.C.S.(C.) stands for the Fellowship of the Royal College of Physicians and Surgeons of Canada.

In theory, any licensed ophthalmologist can perform refractive surgery, but there are surgeons who complete a subspecialty fellowship in this area. In order to use the excimer laser, a short certification course must first be taken.

The Optometrist

Optometrists usually begin their post-secondary training with a four year bachelor of science degree. From there, they enter a school of optometry where they enroll in a four year program. Their training includes a similar study of the basic sciences, including anatomy, physiology, pathology, ocular pharmacology, and optics, in addition to seeing patients. Optometric students spend a significant proportion of time and energy devoted to the refractive sciences, as this constitutes the bulk of a typical optometric practice. Upon successful completion of their program, they are awarded the designation O.D. (Doctor of Optometry). Some optometrists choose to enroll in a one year residency program in a subspecialty such as contact lenses or low vision. More letters, such as F.A.A.O. (Fellow of the American Academy of Optometry), may be awarded to optometrists who demonstrate special interests and abilities.

In the real world, optometrists assess, measure, and diagnose the condition of the eye. In addition, optometrists are involved in ocular health education and research. Traditionally, the role of optometrists has centred around refraction, however they are striving to become more involved the treatment of ocular disease. In some states and provinces, optometrists have been awarded the privilege of prescribing ocular medications.

There are national and regional licensing boards which require the passing of written and oral examinations. The American version is the National Board of Examiners in Optometry and the northern counterpart is the Canadian Examiners in Optometry.

Optometrists are *not* medical doctors.

The Optician

Without opticians, the world would be a hazy place. They are the miracle workers who take an illegible piece of paper, combine it with a fashionable yet sophisticated frame, add just enough tint to highlight the purple in your hair, and end up providing you with a crystal clear, perfectly fit set of glasses.

The Ophthalmic Assistant, Technician, and Medical Technologist

When you walk into an eye doctor's office, often the first person to test your eyes is not the same person whose name appears on the door. Among other things, this individual checks your vision, measures your pupils, puts drops in your eyes, and performs a number of different tests depending on their level of training and experience. The Joint Commission on Allied Health Personnel in Ophthalmology is the certification board which orchestrates a training and evaluation program. There are several levels of certification, ranging from the ophthalmic assistant (basic) to the ophthalmic technician (intermediate) to the ophthalmic medical technologist (advanced). Certification is based on a combination of course requirements, examinations, work experience, and continuing education.

Ophthalmologists and Optometrists
(Similarities and differences at a glance)

	Ophthalmologist	Optometrist
Eye doctors	Yes	Yes
Medical doctors	Yes	No
University degree	M.D./D.O	O.D.
Prescribe glasses, contact lenses	Yes	Yes
Prescribe drugs	Yes	Variable*
Perform surgery	Yes	No
Perform PRK	Yes	No
Perform LASIK, RK, lensectomy	Yes	No
Perform post-laser care	Yes	Yes
Long, difficult word to spell	Yes	Yes

*In some states and provinces, optometrists can prescribe ocular medication.

WHO TO SEE?

For your regular eye care, you can see whomever you wish: your optometrist, your ophthalmologist, your acupuncturist. The important thing is to make an educated decision and to find someone you are comfortable with. It goes back to the premise that the most important determinant of a quality doctor is if they're a quality person. Consequently, there are good ophthalmologists and not so good ones. The same applies to optometrists, football players, and actors. Find someone you like and trust and stick with them.

If you're considering refractive surgery, it's not so easy. Optometrists do not perform surgery. Although it is conceivable that PRK may one day be

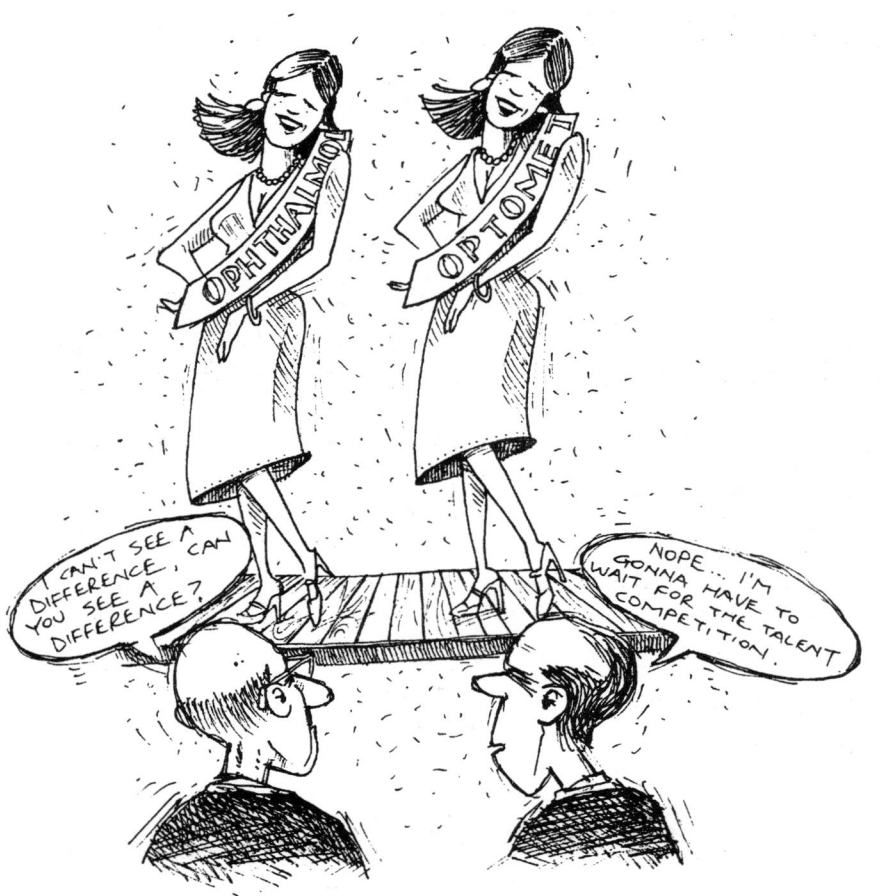

performed by optometrists across the country, their options will likely be restricted. Unless things change radically, optometrists will not be allowed to perform any of the other current treatments, including LASIK, RK, AK, and refractive lensectomy. That means that, both now and in the future, you will likely need an ophthalmologist to perform the actual procedure.

CHOOSING AN OPHTHALMOLOGIST

Yellow Pages were not invented just to torment the color blind. There is a certain uncomfortable randomness in the process, but it is not a bad place to start. Don't be misled by the ads. Size, as always, is not important.

Referrals from your family doctor are often helpful. Often they are aware of the surgeon's reputation within the medical community and they can steer you away from trouble.

Referrals from your optometrist or ophthalmologist (if they do not perform refractive surgery themselves) can be useful. Bear in mind, however, that their recommendations may not be entirely objective. These individuals may be aligned with certain refractive surgeons or laser centres. Their arrangements may include anything from a financial incentive for referring you, to a promise that you will be returned to the referring doctor for post-operative care. Their advice may be good, but it may not be unbiased. Some healthy skepticism may be wise.

Advertisements are becoming more common. Radio, newspapers, and magazines are popular, but television is not far behind. The ads are usually for a certain laser centre or for a specific doctor. Ads are ads and they are probably most useful for getting a name and number.

Word of mouth is another way to get a name. In fact, it is the single most common reason you end up on a doctor's doorstep. Unless your friends and family are shrewd enough to negotiate a financial kickback for referring you, their opinions are unbiased. Your sister's good result is encouraging, but remember, just because the first M & M is red doesn't mean that they all are. Using some or all of these sources, you should develop a list of names. If you feel lucky, throw a dart at your list and you'll have your answer in seconds. If, on the other hand, you decide to exercise your best judgement, then perhaps it is time to do some research.

Some centres offer seminars for prospective patients. Take an evening and attend one or two. Not only will the actual content be helpful, you will also get an idea as to their style. Hard sell, high pressure, or just the facts ma'am. Do they explain the risks as well as the benefits? Are their success rates unbelievably high or frighteningly low? Do everybody's socks match? Attention to detail is paramount.

You probably wouldn't buy a car from the first dealer you meet. Shop around. Make comparisons. Ask good questions. Don't be afraid to let them know that you've done your homework.

Once you've been suitably impressed, make an appointment. They may charge you for the consultation, but consider it an investment. Remember, this is a learning experience and you can walk away at any time.

THE CONSULTATION

Your History

In order to give good advice, your doctor needs to learn about you and your eyes. Whether it involves a face to face interview or a written questionnaire, the content is similar. It is in your best interest to tell the truth, the whole truth, and nothing but the truth.

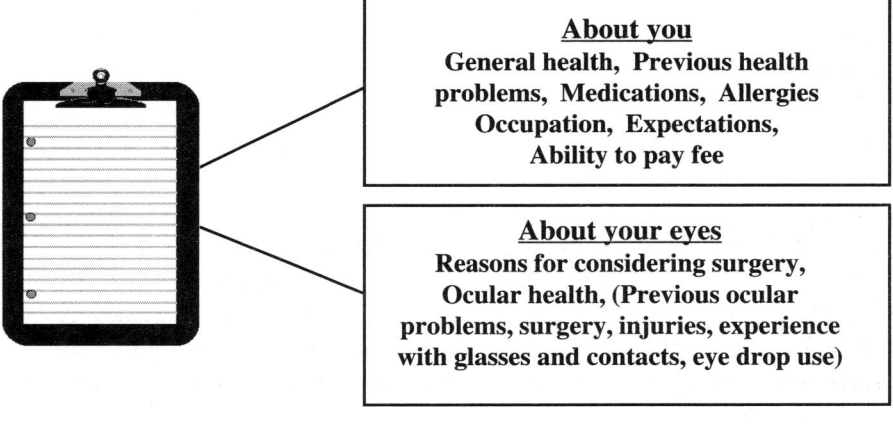

About you
General health, Previous health problems, Medications, Allergies Occupation, Expectations, Ability to pay fee

About your eyes
Reasons for considering surgery, Ocular health, (Previous ocular problems, surgery, injuries, experience with glasses and contacts, eye drop use)

The Examination

In order to determine if you are a good candidate for refractive surgery, a thorough ocular examination should be performed.

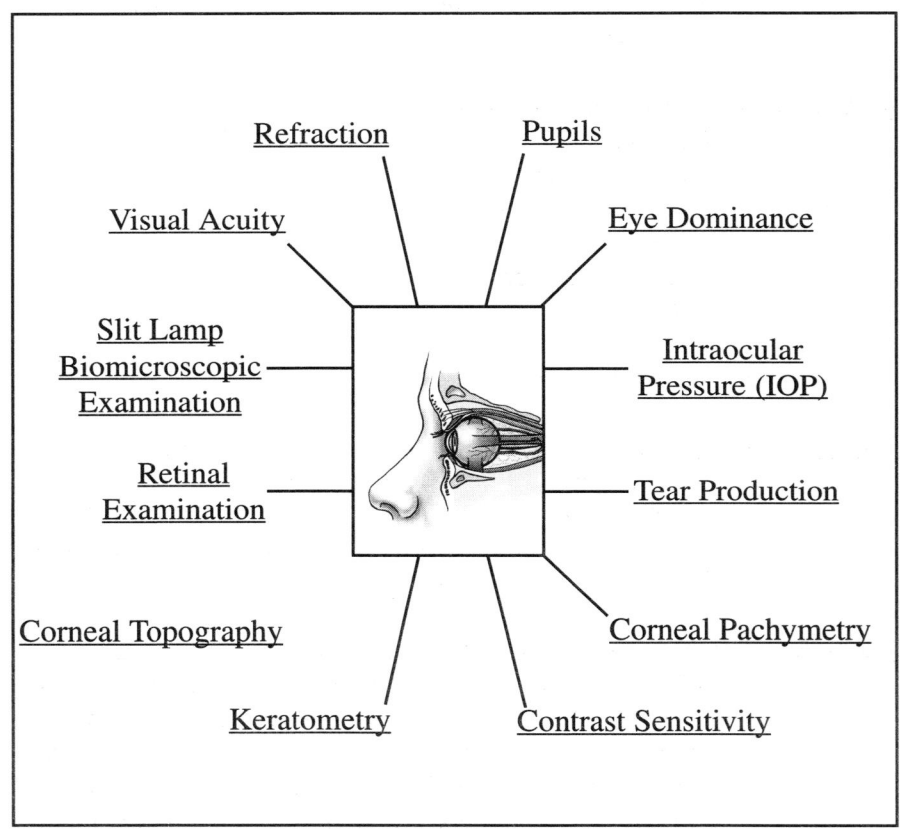

Visual acuity :   -Uncorrected
                 -Best corrected
                 -Corrected
                 -Pinhole
                 -Near

Refraction :   Current - your current prescription
               Manifest - the best prescription which can be obtained
               Cycloplegic - the best prescription which can be obtained
               after the use of dilating drops

Eye dominance

Pupils: Reactivity - abnormal pupillary reactions suggest ocular disease
Size - important in minimizing post-operative glare symptoms

Slit lamp biomicroscopic examination:
Essential routine screening for ocular disease
Lids and lashes
Conjunctiva and Sclera
Cornea
Anterior chamber
Iris
Lens
Anterior vitreous

Intraocular pressure (IOP): A basketball has a certain pressure. If it is rock hard, the pressure is high, compared to a flat basketball which has a low pressure. The equivalent pressure of the eye is known as the intraocular pressure (IOP). Normal IOP is less than 22 mm of mercury.

Tear production: Many people have dry eyes. In fact, many people have difficulty wearing contact lenses for this reason. There is a large spectrum in this condition, ranging from mild to severe. Because eyes which are significantly dry are at risk for post-operative complications, it is important to recognize it early on. The most common way of assessing tear production is the Schirmer's test. After freezing the eye with drops, a piece of special filter paper is placed in the eye. After five minutes, the amount of wetting is measured. Inadequate tear production should be recognized, quantified, and addressed before surgery.

Retinal examination: Individuals who are nearsighted have a higher risk of retinal problems than the general population. The greater the myopia, the greater the risk. Specifically, myopic eyes have an increased chance of developing sight-threatening problems, such as a retinal detachment, over the course of their lifetime. On occasion, tears in the retina may be identified on routine examination and treatment of these areas may prevent potentially catastrophic problems from developing. Because the promise of 20/20 is often the only thing which will lure otherwise healthy people into an ophthalmologists office, this initial consultation may be the first time that a peripheral retinal examination has ever been performed. Dilating drops are instilled and the poor unsuspecting myope is tortured with a disorienting series of bright lights.

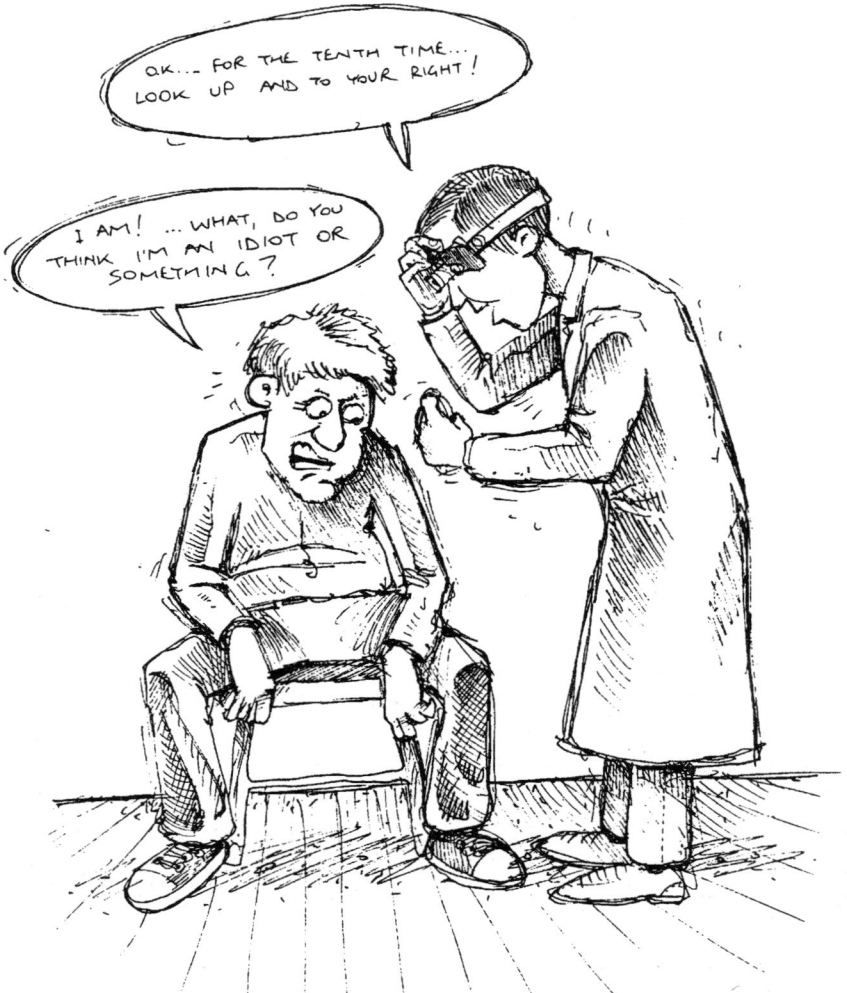

Corneal pachymetry: The thickness of the cornea is measured by a pachymeter. This information is required to plan surgical depths.

Corneal topography: The result of recent technological advances, corneal topography is rapidly becoming a vital pre-operative, as well as post-operative test. It is analogous to topographical maps of the earth, which represent areas of hills and valleys using linear contours. The corneal version plots the steepness of the entire corneal surface, highlighting areas of astigmatism and asymmetry. The results are displayed in a color coded picture which can be used to plan treatment or assess surgical outcomes.

Keratometry: This test measures diopteric power of the cornea, which is necessary in planning surgery.

Contrast sensitivity: Instead of measuring black on white acuity, this is a more sensitive vision test which involves various shades of grey.

The Discussion

By integrating all of these morsels of information, the surgeon can piece together a complete picture of your eyes. This ensuing discussion is the most critical part of the initial consultation.

General strategies

Image isn't everything. Different car salesmen have different styles. Doctors are the same. Some will be a little over the top, calling you an "ideal candidate" with an "excellent prognosis". Surgery will, of course, be "highly recommended". Others will simply present you with the facts and allow you to make the decision on your own. Getting a "recommendation" is like pulling teeth. The bottom line is that if you like the car, yet you hate the salesman's tie, you should probably still buy the car. Style is not important.

Content is everything. Listen to what the surgeon has to say. Probably a majority of your questions will be answered. Save up your questions until the end, but interrupt if you don't understand something. Don't be afraid to take notes, or pull out a list of questions. Do not feel rushed or pressured. It is not your job to worry about the waiting room full of people. Your eyes should be your only concern.

Bring someone with you. A friend or a family member is often helpful. Two brains and memories are better than one, and a little moral support can't hurt. Usually just one, though. Three's a crowd and you don't want to get lost in the background.

Be careful with numbers. Do not be satisfied with terms like "excellent" and "most". Compare with the numbers in this book and compare with other surgeons. There's a huge difference between 80% of people seeing 20/20 post-operatively, and 90%. In fairness to the surgeon, numbers are often not exact. If you are a 22 year old white female with a refractive error of -4.50-2.25 X 120, who happens to be a rigid contact lens wearer and a left-handed bowler, what is your chance of success? Unless your surgeon recently performed surgery on your other four quintuplet siblings, nobody knows exactly. Using a combination of experience and knowledge, and extrapolating from results in similar patients, reasonable ballpark figures can be offered. Remember, though, interpretation of the numbers is tricky. A single study can demonstrate that ninety-five percent of patients were satisfied with the results, but only five percent would do it all over again. Statistics are notoriously confusing and to make matters worse, all scientific studies are not created equal. The design of the experiments, not to mention the quality of the data and analysis, influences the final numbers. Although it may take a Master's degree to comprehend all of the details, the take home message is that if it seems too good to be true, it might just be.

Do your homework. Instead of just kicking the tires and professing your ignorance, read books, surf the Net, and talk to people. Become comfortable using terms like best-corrected and uncorrected. Make your surgeon talk to you, not down to you. You will get a clearer picture of the expected results.

Listen, look, and learn. A great deal of information is available to the curious. Is the waiting room full or empty? Are people in the waiting room happy? Are the support staff wearing glasses? Is the surgeon? (If so, ask

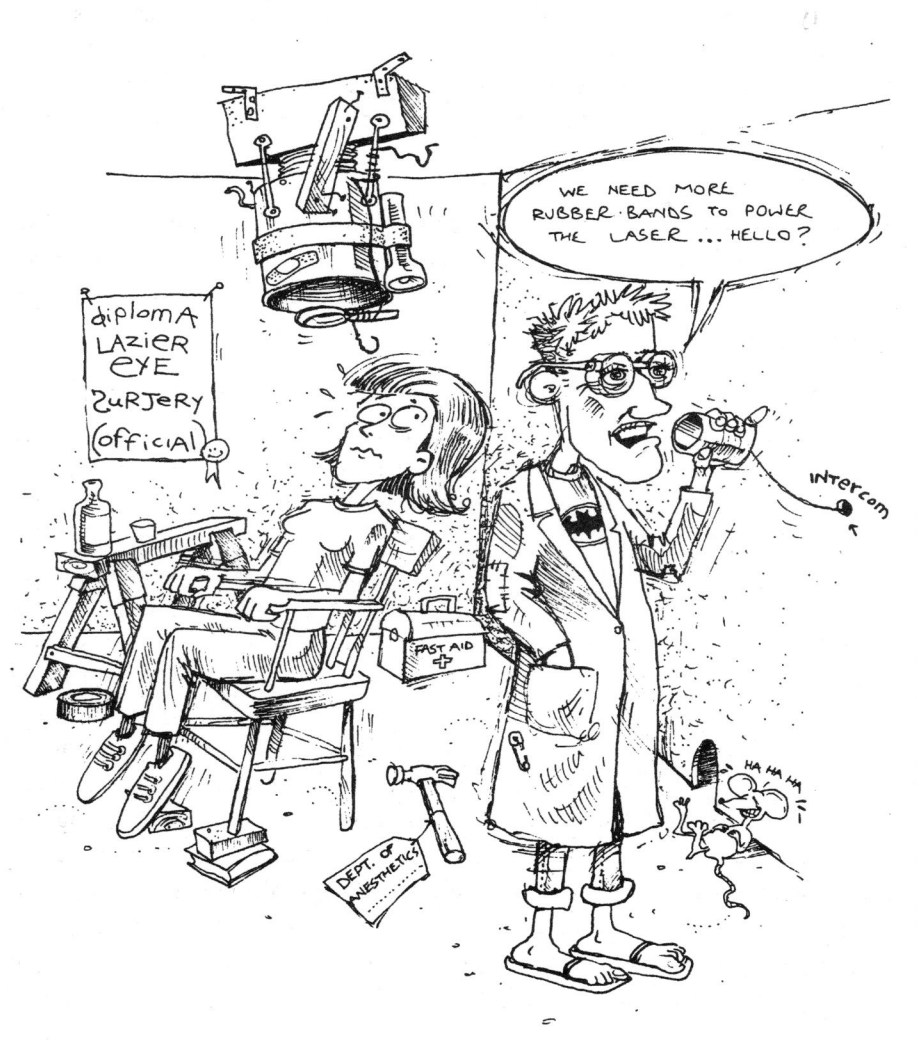

why.) Are their telephones rotary or touch-tone? Are the diplomas on the wall from the ACME School of Medicine? None of these are important in themselves, but they can help fill in the blanks.

Get specific answers to specific questions.

Questions To Ask Your Doctor

About the Doctor

What are your qualifications?
(Board-eligible, board certified fellowship
trained, FRCS(C)).

What kind of experience have you had?
(RK vs PRK vs LASIK.)

How many cases have you done? (There is no exact cutoff,
but there is a learning curve. This is one situation where
being #1 is not necessarily a good thing.)

Who will be doing my surgery? (Just because you go to
Dr. X's laser centre doesn't mean that Dr. X will be
the one operating.)

About the Procedure

Would I be a good candidate for refractive surgery?
(Better than asking "should I have surgery?")

Which procedure would you recommend?
(And why?)

What are the alternatives?
(Specifically, is LASIK being considered, and if not, why not?)

Should I have both eyes done?
(Should monovision be considered?)

Is there any reason why I should not have both eyes
done on the same day?

Questions about the Post-Operative Course

How much pain will I have? (Not the most brilliant question in the world, but one you have to ask! And it gives the doctor a chance to reassure you that his or her way is virtually pain-free.)

Which drops do you routinely prescribe?

How long will I be taking them?
(Expect a range, eg. one month to six months)

Do you insert a bandage contact lens post-operatively?
(Usually used after PRK, but not LASIK)

Should I plan on taking time off work?
(If so, how long?)

When are follow-up appointments scheduled?
(Close, regular follow-up is essential)

Is there someone available for post-operative emergencies?
(24 hours/seven days?)

Questions about Success Rates

What is the chance that I will see 20/20 uncorrected post-operatively?

What is the chance that I will see 20/40 (usual driving standard) uncorrected post-operatively?

What is the chance that I will need glasses or contacts post-operatively?

What is the chance that I will need to have a second or third procedure?

What percentage of your patients are happy that they have had it done? (Some laser centres keep track of these statistics through post-operative surveys)

What percentage of your patients would do it all over again or recommend it to a friend?

Questions about Risks and Complications

What is the chance that my best-corrected vision will deteriorate?

What is the chance that my uncorrected vision will deteriorate?

Is there anything about my eyes that puts me at a higher risk of complications than the general population?
(Better to find out now.)

Questions about Money

How much? (If money is a significant issue, ask about differences between RK, PRK, and LASIK)

What is included in the fee?

What is not included in the fee?

Is it less expensive to have both eyes done together (or close together)?

Is there a charge for touch-ups?

Do you have a financing plan/accept credit cards?

Are there group discounts? (Friends, family, corporate)

The specifics of the discussion will depend on you and your eyes. One particular issue is worth examining in detail, *the second eye.*

THE SECOND EYE

If?

Most people who choose to have a refractive procedure elect to have both eyes done.

Advantages: Throw away the glasses (ideally)
Little or no imbalance between eyes
Good depth perception

Disadvantages: Cost
Loss of potentially helpful difference between eyes (see *Monovision* section this chapter)

When?

If you want both eyes done, there are two possibilities. Now or later. Now means same day or simultaneous bilateral surgery. That is, both eyes are operated on at the same time. Later, for all intents and purposes, means not now.

Simultaneous Bilateral Surgery

Advantages: *Getting it over with*. The pain, the visual disturbance, the stress. Why go through it twice if you can get away with only once?

No comparison. Often, people who have simultaneous bilateral surgery are happier with the result. They are not constantly making comparisons between the operated and unoperated eyes.

No anisometropia. Individuals who are intolerant of contact lenses may be spared the imbalance associated with two different spectacle lenses.

Disadvantages: *Complications*. In the unlikely event that you suffer a complication, you may wish that you had only one eye

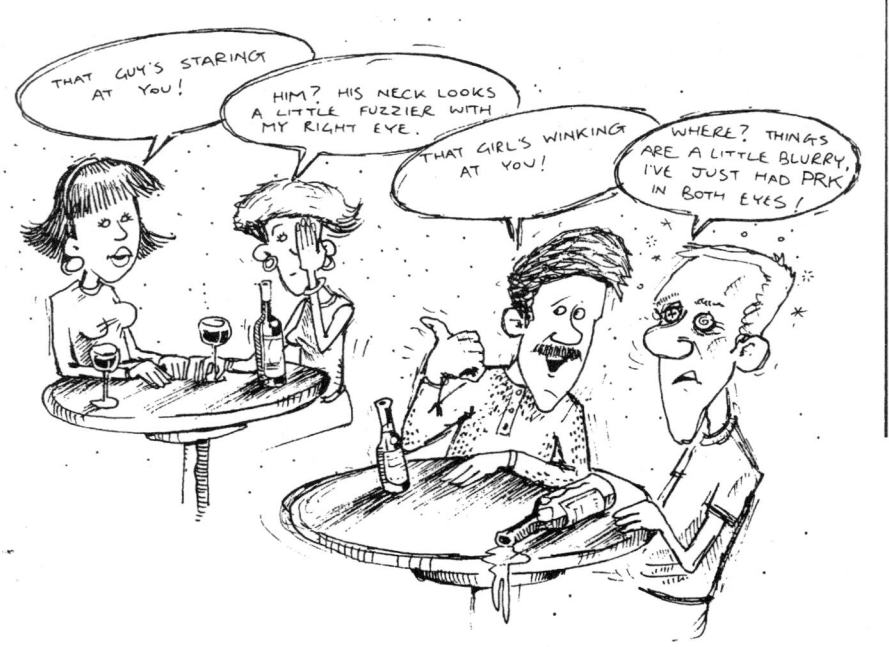

done. A blinding infection (exceedingly rare) in one eye is bad. In both eyes (never yet seen to our knowledge), it would be worse. Much worse. There are doctors out there who refuse to perform bilateral surgery because of this complication alone.

Not approved. The American Food and Drug Administration (FDA) has not approved bilateral simultaneous surgery. There recommendation is a minimum of three months between eyes. Just because it isn't approved, however, doesn't mean that it isn't a reasonable option.

Visual impairment. Until the eyes heal, you will have trouble seeing. That means no driving, working, or operating heavy machinery until at least one of the eyes improves sufficiently. If you're considering PRK, that could take weeks.

No learning effect. If one eye is done first, your surgeon can learn from the response. Remember, everyone heals differently. If your first eye is overcorrected, compensatory adjustments can be made to the second eye. If both eyes are done together, unless you have three eyes, this learning effect is wasted. This learning effect is not a hundred percent reliable, however. Surgeons have found that individual and environmental variations may account for a different response in the second eye, even if the identical treatment was performed.

Testing the waters. There are people who have the procedure on one eye and are unhappy, for whatever reason, with the result. At least you retain the option to back out of the second eye.

Which?

If both eyes are operated on at the same sitting, it doesn't matter which one is done first. It's like asking which twin is older? If, however, you've decided on one eye at a time, which eye should be the first? The left or the right? The better or the worse? The blue or the brown?

In order to answer that question, we need to understand the concept of dominance. One of your eyes is the *dominant* eye and the other one is called, big surprise, the *non-dominant* eye. How do you know which is which? To answer that question, you will need some high tech equipment. A piece of paper with a small hole will do the trick. Pick a small object across the room, perhaps a doorknob or a light switch. Now lift up the paper with both hands, keeping it at arms length. Looking through the hole, identify the object. Slowly bring the paper toward you, watching the object the entire time. When the paper comes close to your face, you will find that you were using only one eye to see the object. Whichever eye has the hole in front of it is your dominant eye.

Sometimes, the question of dominance is clear cut. In other people, it is difficult to tell, in which case the eyes may be termed co-dominant.

The issue of dominance is important for a couple of reasons.

Timing of surgery

If the two eyes are significantly different, the one with the greater refractive error or worse best-corrected visual acuity is done first if simultaneous surgery is not being performed. If the two eyes are similar, the non-dominant eye is usually done first. This way, any learning effect can be applied to the procedure on the better, dominant eye. If the eyes are co-dominant and the two eyes are identical, the decision is made on a purely scientific basis: heads is right and tails is left.

Monovision

This concept was explored earlier in the section on contact lenses. The idea remains the same in this context. One eye is corrected for near and the other eye is corrected for distance. This technique is useful for patients in their forties and older who are presbyopic. (Younger patients retain good accommodative power in their lenses which enables them to focus up close unassisted.) If both eyes are corrected for 20/20 in the distance, reading glasses will be necessary to compensate for the insufficient accommodative reserve. Monovision aims to leave one eye slightly myopic, usually around -1 D, to allow clearer near vision with that eye. Assuming that the difference between the two eyes is not too great, this can be a valuable method of reducing the dependence on reading glasses. Typically, if monovision is desired, the dominant eye will be corrected for distance and the non-dominant eye for near.

Monovision may be useful in other scenarios as well. If you're 35 years old and have a prescription of -3 D in both eyes, you would likely elect to have both eyes targeted for full correction. If the first eye is left with mild residual myopia, monovision becomes an acceptable alternative to retreatment. Instead of trying to eliminate the -1 D refractive error with enhancement surgery, it may be worthwhile leaving it as is, operating on the other eye, and trying to adapt to and enjoy the long-term benefits of monovision. Sooner or later, the presbyopic pixie will sprinkle dust in your eyes, and you will be ready and waiting.

Similarly, if your right eye has a refractive error of -3 D and your left eye is a -1 D, it may be worth operating on only the right. This way, you can keep the mildly myopic left eye as your ace in the hole for when that pixie comes to get you.

The primary advantage to monovision is the freedom from reading glasses when you reach the presbyopic age group. This is particularly helpful for people such as teachers, musicians, and public speakers, who need to keep switching their focus from near to far.

There are disadvantages to monovision. Decreased depth perception may result from the difference between the two eyes. In certain situations where the "distance" eye is covered, the image from the "near" eye may seem somewhat blurred when you look far away.

Will I need to wear glasses after refractive surgery?

The answer to that big question is a definitive no...unless...

Unless the results of surgery are not perfect. Surgical success is customarily assessed in terms of refraction and vision. Check the percentages in the upcoming chapters for your specific chances. 20/40 is the usual driving standard. If 95% of people with your refractive error achieve 20/40 uncorrected, you have a pretty good chance of being able to drive legally without glasses. The numbers do not tell the whole story, however. If you are 20/40 uncorrected, you may *choose* to wear glasses for driving and other special activities, if you feel that it helps. Still, most people with this level of vision find that they can perform most basic daily activities without glasses. Curiously, there are people with worse vision who are happy without glasses. It comes down to the amount of improvement you get with glasses, and whether or not you feel this makes a significant difference to you. Having said that, if your post-operative refraction is plano in both eyes, and your uncorrected vision is 20/20, chances are you won't need glasses. Unless.

Unless you're over forty and presbyopic, in which case your eye's natural accommodative ability is not what it used to be. This means that if you require no distance prescription post-operatively, you will either need reading glasses or longer arms. If you were hyperopic before the surgery, reading glasses may be familiar to you. If you were myopic pre-operatively, you may have been taking advantage of your myopia to avoid reading glasses. When your myopia is surgically removed, your built in reading glasses disappear with it. There is one special situation worth mentioning. If you are over forty and choose *monovision,* you may be able to get away without reading glasses for some near activities. If you're less than forty, you can breathe a sigh of relief. You're all right for now, but sooner or later, mother nature will catch up to you and slip a set of reading glasses in your pocket. For the moment, anyway, you may be able to get away without them. Unless.

Unless you need or choose to have a cataract extraction or refractive lensectomy. These procedures usually leave you without any natural accommodation, so reading glasses are required post-operatively. With PRK, LASIK, and RK, your accommodation is preserved so glasses may not be necessary. Unless.

Unless you cannot see as well as you need to. There are people who see 20/ 40 uncorrected, who meet the driving requirements, but who refuse to drive without glasses. They do not feel safe behind the wheel. This phenomenon occurs more often at night, and is a matter of personal preference. Whether you wear glasses all the time or only part of the time, is completely up to you. If you feel that things are clearer with glasses on, and that you need to see better, wearing glasses is the answer. Or if you'd rather not, don't. Unless.

Unless you participate in dangerous sports. Safety glasses are recommended for eye-threatening sports, especially in an eye which has had RK.

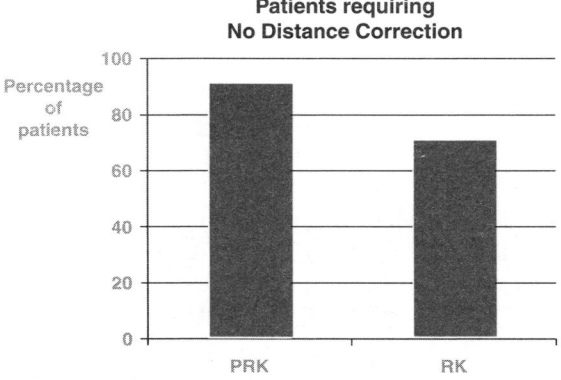

Patients requiring No Distance Correction

PART TWO

THE SURGICAL TREATMENT OF MYOPIA

5

PHOTO REFACTIVE KERATECTOMY (PRK)

THE LASER

What is a Laser?

LASER stands for Light Amplification by Stimulated Emission of Radiation. The first word is a good place to begin. A laser is a light. Not a light like the one in your living room, but a special kind of light. It has unique qualities.

> Monochromaticity - A laser has only one wavelength or color. A regular light bulb has a range of wavelengths.
>
> Directionality - A laser has a narrow beam which does not diverge. Compare a laser pointer with a regular flashlight.
>
> Intensity - A laser is an extremely powerful light. A simple laser can produce light which is a hundred times more intense than sunlight.

These properties make the laser useful in light shows, war games, and incidentally, health care. Within medicine, lasers were first adapted for eye surgery.

The Excimer Laser

Lasers are differentiated from each other by the wavelength of their light beam. A laser generated from krypton gas produces light with a wavelength of 647 nanometers (nm). This wavelength falls within the visible spectrum of electromagnetic radiation and is seen as red. An argon laser which is used in retinal surgery has a wavelength of 514 nm and is green. A holmium:YAG laser with a wavelength of 2.13 micrometres is useful in the treatment of hyperopia.

The *excimer* laser uses a combination of argon and fluoride gases to produce radiation in the ultraviolet range (193nm) which is invisible to the naked eye. This laser light has the ability to break molecular bonds in a process called *photoablation*. In 1983, it was first realized that this laser could be useful for corneal surgery. Why? Because this laser was different. Unlike other lasers, the excimer had the ability to remove corneal tissue with a high degree of precision, and equally important, without causing thermal damage to the remaining tissue. Sculpting of the cornea entered into the realm of possibility.

It is difficult, yet desirable, to comprehend the degree of precision exhibited by the excimer laser. A millimetre is one thousandth of a metre or four hundredths of an inch. A micron, or micrometre, is one thousandth of a millimetre. That is, one millionth of a metre. For the sake of comparison, a potato chip is about 500 microns thick, a human hair is about 50 microns thick and a single red blood cell is seven microns in diameter. The excimer laser has the ability to sculpt the cornea within *a fraction of a micron*. Advocates of laser surgery point out that the steadiest hands in the world cannot even approach that level of surgical precision.

There are other kinds of lasers on the horizon which act in a similar fashion to the excimer. The light from these *solid state* lasers is produced from a crystal, whereas the excimer beam is created from a gas. Technically, solid state lasers are not excimer lasers, but for the purposes of this book they will be considered interchangeable.

Which laser is the best?

There are several different excimer lasers being used today and that number is growing quickly. Just like in the automobile industry, new models are always in the pipeline, as are refinements of current machines. Each laser system is complicated and each has its own unique twists, advantages, and disadvantages. There is probably one question on your mind. Which laser is the best?

Which car is the best? Suppose that you've decided to buy a new car, but know very little about mechanics. And just to make sure the analogy is fair, assume that money is not an issue. Pretend this is fantasyland. You can have any car you want. Which car would you choose? What is the right answer? Is there a right answer? What is your answer? If you decided on a black Porsche 911, is that any better than a white Mercedes 550 SL? Or a red Dodge Viper? Or a black Hummer? The answer is that there is no right answer. There's good and bad in each vehicle. The choice depends on you, the driver.

Now suppose you won't be doing the driving. (If you can afford these cars, surely you can afford a chauffeur.) You're just a terrified passenger who needs to get from point A to point B. Now what car would you choose. To make that decision, it is probably not necessary to know the gear ratios or the warranty package. It is important to feel comfortable, however, and it is important to know that your driver is comfortable with their machine. It would be reassuring to know that the vehicle is relatively new and well maintained, and that previous passengers have been happy with their journey. Beyond that, the details are not very important. The fortunate fact is that most cars will get you where you need to go. Consequently, your time may be better spent picking the right chauffeur. The same principles apply to lasers.

Having said that, it is still in your best interests to know about the options on the market. In general, there are the first generation lasers, which are the grandfathers in the field. The newer second and third generation machines are somewhat more sophisticated.

In terms of the hardware, there are *diaphragm* delivery systems which shoot the laser in a large enough spot to cover the entire treatment zone. *Scanning* delivery systems use a small-area beam which oscillates back and forth across the treatment zone, ablating tissue layer by layer. Eye tracking devices are available in newer models to reduce the risk of decentration.

Software options include algorithms for myopia, hyperopia, and astigmatism, as well as special modifications known as *pretreatment, multizone,* and *multipass* which were designed to improve the outcome.

Used Lasers

If used cars are resold, what happens to used lasers? They, too, are resold. Not everyone can afford a brand new machine. Is this a problem? That depends. Is a 1997 BMW much different from a 1996 model? Probably not, but a 2006 machine may be much different than a 1996 version. Although a decision should not be made on age alone, all things being equal, perhaps a new laser is preferable to an older model. The same thing applies to cars, computers, and for a few people, spouses. Still, when making an airline reservation, you do not usually ask about the age of your airplane. You rely on people who know about these things to make responsible decisions. Once again, it comes down to confidence in the surgeon, not only to perform surgery, but also to select a safe, effective laser.

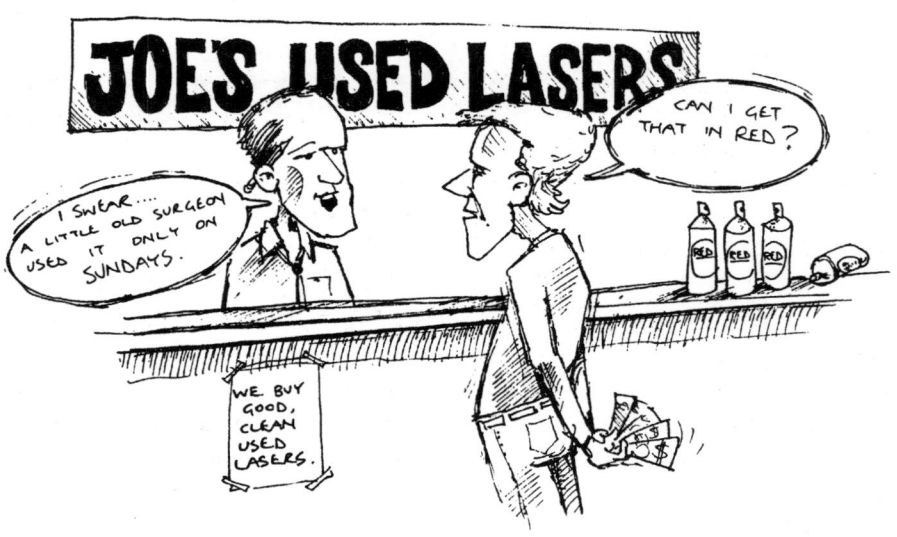

PHOTO REFRACTIVE KERATECTOMY (PRK)

The Road to 1997

The ophthalmic world has been hard at work on PRK since the idea first appeared in 1983. Studies were initially performed in cadaver and rabbit eyes, where the effects of the laser were examined under an electron microscope. In 1984, experimentation on monkeys was conducted and the results were encouraging. Human studies were then initiated, with the first actual procedures being performed on blind eyes in 1987. With optimism, researchers began sighted human experimentation. Increasing numbers of patients were enrolled in large multi-centre trials, designed to document the safety and efficacy of PRK. Finally, in October, 1995, the American Food and Drug Administration (FDA) approved the first excimer laser for use in PRK in the United States.

While the American ophthalmologic community was awaiting FDA approval, the rest of the world was continuing onward. Not bound by U.S. regulations, other countries performed PRK by the thousands. European, South American, Australian, and Canadian ophthalmologists became world leaders in the field. By the time PRK had been approved in the U.S., surgeons had performed in excess of one million PRK procedures worldwide. Internationally, surgeons were not just operating, they were learning. Risks and benefits, strategies and algorithms, theories and practice, nuances and intricacies were all explored. From this experience, modifications were made, not only to surgical technique, but also to the lasers themselves. A whole new procedure, LASIK, (see Chapter 6) was conceived, developed, attempted, and evaluated.

Laser eye surgery is not the same animal it was five years ago. Or even one year ago. Things are changing and, hopefully, improving quickly. The first lasers which appeared on the market are already somewhat antiquated. The original techniques are already demonstrating their imperfections. Tomorrow is anybody's guess.

Is PRK for you?

Technically speaking, PRK can be performed on just about anybody. And if you look hard enough, and are willing to travel to the farthest corners of the world, you will probably find someone who will perform PRK on you. The question is, is it a good idea.

The FDA is the regulatory board for new medical devices in the United States. Not only do they approve a piece of equipment, they also provide indications for its use. For example, if they were to approve a baseball bat for the treatment of a headache, they would detail the nature, severity, and duration of the headache for which the bat should be used, in addition to the number of times daily it should be swung at the head. Furthermore, each particular piece of equipment must receive its own approval for its own indications. Just because a Homerama baseball bat is to be swung twice a day for migraines doesn't mean that a Strikeout bat can't be approved for use in tension headaches four times a day.

The first laser to get the thumbs up was manufactured by Summit Technology Inc.. In Oct, 1995 the FDA approved it for PRK use. This was followed by the VISX Inc. laser a few months later. The initial approval was for a subset of individuals, eyes, and procedures which met certain conditions, including age, refractive error, and treatment zone size.

Other laser manufacturers are hot on the trail and a number of lasers are expected to obtain FDA approval in short order.

What does this mean?: If you fulfil all of the criteria and you'd like to have PRK, everything is straightforward. Step right up, sign the papers, pay your money, and the procedure will be scheduled before you can say twenty-twenty.

What if you do not fall into the "approved" category? Say you're one of the 30% of Americans who have more than the approved 1.5 D of astigmatism or that you're a -8 D myope, which is outside the range of current PRK approval. Or say you've done some homework and decided that you'd prefer LASIK (see Chapter 6) over PRK. Now what? If you live in Canada, it's no big deal. Canadian ophthalmologists do not have to answer to the American FDA. If you and your Canadian surgeon believe that LASIK is right for you, nothing will stop you.

If you live in the U.S., things are a little confusing. There is an ongoing debate between refractive surgeons and the FDA. The FDA can approve a laser for use in certain conditions, but in theory, it is up to the doctors to use their expertise to make the final decision. Still, the FDA prefers doctors to use the laser only for the approved indications. They asked nicely for the surgeons to comply, however some surgeons went ahead and began using their lasers for these "off-label" indications. The doctors' rationale was that their patients should have access to the best care possible. How, argued the physicians, could they in good conscience, refuse treatment to a -8 D myope? Or how could they refuse to perform LASIK if they believed it to be a superior procedure to PRK? If the current medical literature supports new forms of treatment, they have an obligation to offer these to their patients, regardless of FDA approval. The FDA, together with the medical community and the laser manufacturers, are in the process of trying to sort out the matter. For the time being, off-label deployment of the excimer label is being discouraged outside of investigational use. The discussion, however, is ongoing, with both sides claiming and believing that they have your best interests in mind. How it will end in your neighborhood, nobody knows. Generalizations and predictions are dangerous. The best advice is, if you fall outside of the approved parameters for treatment, take a look around. See if somebody is willing and able to help you.

If you cannot find an American surgeon willing to perform PRK on your -8 D myopia, you might decide to participate in a study. Prior to its approval in certain categories, PRK was being performed on thousands of American patients. The research data had to come from somewhere. Right now, there are FDA trials underway for PRK in higher myopes, myopes with astigmatism, and for larger treatment zones. Centres who are interested in performing such procedures apply for an *Investigational Device Exemption* which permits them to perform studies. LASIK is also being studied on American soil, so you may not necessarily need to leave the country to undergo this treatment.

If you cannot find a surgeon in your area who can help, you may wish to combine laser eye surgery with a Canadian ski vacation or a South American scuba diving adventure. Alternatively, you can wait until the FDA has approved the excimer for your specific requirements.

Interestingly, although one does not necessarily need FDA approval to perform the procedure, an ophthalmologist cannot "market or promote" surgery which does not conform to the FDA's guidelines. For this reason, you may not have seen the term LASIK in American ads.

Contraindications

PRK should not be performed, or performed with caution, in people who have certain *contraindications:*

> Mental health - PRK should be avoided in patients if they or their legal guardians are unable to understand fully the potential risks and benefits of the procedure.

> General health - Patients should be in good health without medical problems which could potentially interfere with wound healing. PRK should be avoided in patients with the following:

>> Pregnancy/Nursing - Hormonal changes may interfere with normal wound healing.
>> Impaired immunity (eg. AIDS, steroid use)
>> Autoimmune diseases (eg. rheumatoid arthritis)
>> Diabetes mellitus - Wound healing may be abnormal.

> Ocular health - PRK should be avoided in patients with any significant ocular disease, and specifically, the following:

> One functional eye - If the best-corrected vision in one eye is worse than 20/40, the procedure should possibly not be done. The potential risk is greater than the potential benefit. Operating on the one good eye may be too risky, whereas it may not be worth treating the bad eye because of limited potential benefit.

> Corneal disease - (eg. keratoconus, severe dry eye, herpes simplex/zoster keratitis)

> Unstable refractive error - The refraction should be stable for at least six months.

> Previous eye surgery

PREPARING FOR PRK

If, after the initial consultation, you and your surgeon feel that you would like to proceed with PRK, surgery may be scheduled.

Preparing the patient

Informed consent: Prior to any surgical procedure, you must provide your physician with your *informed consent*. Those two innocent words, when joined together in a medical setting, have inspired countless definitions and endless debates. The essence, however, is simple. If you wish to undergo a procedure, you must be aware of its risks, benefits, and alternatives. Only then is it truly an *informed* consent. This is especially important in refractive surgery because of the elective nature of the procedure. Nobody is making you have the procedure, and unlike heart surgery, the risks to *not* having surgery are minimal.

Usually, doctors obtain informed consent by explaining the procedure, answering your questions, and having you sign a consent form. Some ophthalmologists are taking the issue one step further. Not only do they ask you to review the information, but they also insist that you demonstrate your understanding of the procedure and its limitations. You may be given a short test (gasp!) to confirm your comprehension.

PRK Consent Form Questionnaire

**Directions: Please answer the following True/False questions
to assure us that you understand the information discussed with you.**

True	False	
T	F	1. PRK is a completely safe surgical procedure and is not subject to risks associated with other types of surgery.
T	F	2. It may take several weeks after surgery before I have functional vision
T	F	3. There is a chance my eye may regress to being almost as nearsighted as before the surgery.

T   F   4. I may experience halos around lights at night after the surgery.

T   F   5. Halos and glare always go away with time.

T   F   6. Infection occurs very rarely, but if it does, it could lead to loss of vision and corneal scarring.

T   F   7. The cornea is at risk for infection for up to three months post-operatively.

T   F   8. I may be taking eye drops for several weeks or months following the surgery.

T   F   9. My eye will be completely healed and stable by three months post-operatively.

T   F   10. Haze is part of the natural healing process of my eye and does not usually affect the vision.

T   F   11. More significant haze can develop that may affect the vision and may require further treatment.

T   F   12. If my cornea heals in an irregular fashion, I can always wear glasses or contact lenses to correct my vision to 20/20.

T   F   13. Monovision is a situation that works best for people under the age of forty.

T   F   14. Monovision means having one eye slightly nearsighted to read with and the other eye corrected for distance.

T   F   15. If I have a good surgical result and can see 20 20 in the distance, I will eventually require reading glasses for near work.

T   F   16. The purpose of refractive surgery is to totally eliminate glasses for all activities.

T	F	17. A small percentage of people will have significant discomfort in the first 48 hours.
T	F	18. PRK is not the only alternative to reduce or eliminate a refractive error.
T	F	19. The majority of PRK patients see well enough that they do not wear distance corrective lenses after the surgery.
T	F	20. My eyes may be sensitive to light and I may experience some increased glare after surgery.

Answers

1. False   No surgery is completely safe. There are always risks, however they are minimal with PRK.

2. True   Your vision may be quite blurry for the first few weeks to months after surgery, but it should gradually improve.

3. True   Some patients have a stronger than normal healing response causing the eye to regress. A small number of patients may experience a large amount of regression.

4. True   Halos at night are usually caused by the pupil dilating larger than the treated zone. This improves with time for most patients.

5. False   A small number of patients are bothered by halos indefinitely. This can interfere with night driving.

6. True   The risk of infection is very minimal but is a possibility. If you were to develop an infection, it could be vision threatening.

7. False   The risk of infection is only until the surface layer of the cornea, the epithelium, is healed over and intact. This usually occurs within a few days.

8. True   You will be put on anti-inflammatory drops after your epithelium has healed over. You may be taking them for months after your surgery.

9. False   While most patients are quite stable by three months post operatively, some patients continue to show changes in their refraction for longer periods of time.

10. True   Almost all patients will develop a slight haze of the cornel as a normal healing response. Most often, the patient is not aware of it and it does not affect the vision.

11. True   A small number of patients can develop more significant haze that can affect vision. This is due to a stronger than normal healing response and may require further treatment.

12. False   Irregular corneal healing is a condition which may cause reduction in vision. It occurs in a small number of people and it is not always treatable with glasses, contact lenses, or surgery.

13. False   Most people under age forty will not appreciate the benefits of monovision as they have probably not yet begun to experience difficulties with near vision.

14. True   As a person ages, the lens of his/her eye becomes harder and less able to focus for near vision. Therefore, having one eye nearsighted will enable the patient to read with that eye and to use the other eye for distance.

15. True   If both eyes are corrected well to see in the distance, I will still require reading glasses as presbyopia sets in.

16. False   The purpose of refractive surgery is to make patients less dependent on glasses or contact lenses, and to provide more functional vision. Perfect vision without glasses cannot be guaranteed. You may require glasses for

certain activities (such as night driving or reading) post operatively.

17. True   While most patients experience only a slight discomfort (a scratchy, sandy sensation), a small number of patients can experience more significant discomfort in the first two days following surgery.

18. True   PRK is not the only alternative to correct your refractive error.

19. True   The majority of PRK patients see well enough that they do not require corrective lenses for distance after surgery.

20. True   Your eyes may be sensitive to light and you may experience some glare post-operatively.

Contact lens wear: Because a contact lens rests on the surface of the eye itself, your cornea may be directly affected. Consequently, contact lenses can distort the results of pre-operative tests. In order to ensure that any contact lens effect is minimized, you should discontinue them prior to testing. Daily wear soft contact lenses have the least impact on the cornea, and they should be stopped one to two weeks before surgery. Extended wear and rigid lenses have a greater effect and they should not be worn for four to six weeks pre-operatively. For some contact lens wearers, this requirement is like a prison sentence. The use of disposable lenses in the interim, although not ideal for the surgeon or the patient, may be the best compromise.

The important concept here is stability. In order to make sure that your cornea receives the appropriate amount of treatment, your eye should not be changing. Refractions and corneal topography should be repeated until your surgeon is satisfied that stability has been achieved.

Drops, tears, and scrubs: It is important to optimize the function of the eyes before surgery. If your eyes are dry, they should be lubricated. If that is inadequate, tear loss may be prevented by using special drainage plugs. On the day of surgery, makeup should not be worn. Pre-operatively, your face is washed with an antiseptic solution. Antibiotic and topical anaesthetic drops make your eyes clean and comfortable.

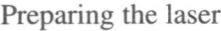

Preparing the laser

At the risk of sparking a heated debate on the existence of artificial intelligence, it is a known fact that a computer cannot think. In this context, that means that the laser machine must be told what to do. When given the appropriate instructions, it performs its task with precision and diligence. But before the computer can help you, it needs to know a little bit about your eye.

It has been said that the most important part of the entire PRK procedure takes place before the surgeon enters the laser suite. In a back room perhaps, or at home the night before, or maybe even in the cafeteria at lunchtime, the surgeon must decide on your treatment parameters. After reviewing your chart in an energy-intensive, brain-taxing sit-down-think, a few numbers emerge. This data is input into the laser and will, in large part, determine the outcome of the surgery.

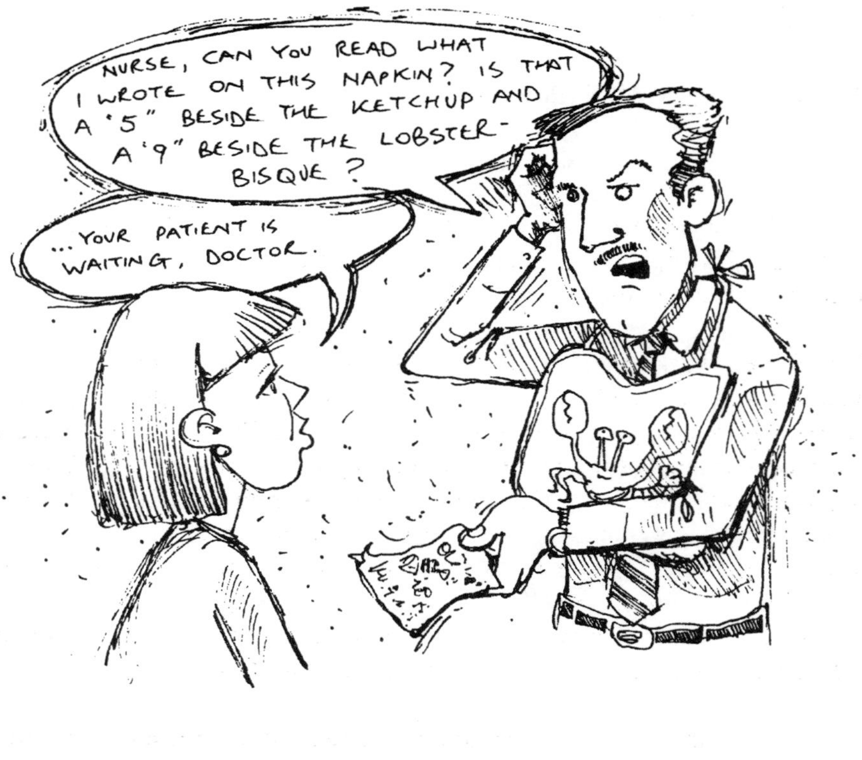

One of the variables which requires attention is the optical zone size. There are advantages to a large zone. Halos, as will soon be described, may occur if the pupil is larger than the treatment zone. So why not just perform a large zone treatment on everybody? Well, there are limits. In general, the larger the treatment zone, the deeper the laser treatment will be. Because the cornea does not like to be invaded to great depths, PRK is best confined to its front third. In addition, there are individual variations in pupil size and corneal diameter. Taking into account these factors, a balance must be struck between the size and depth of the treatment zone.

Once the laser knows what to do, it is important to make sure that it can, in fact, do the job. Calibration of the laser, therefore, is an essential part of the pre-operative preparation. The amount of energy (fluence) and the pattern of its distribution (homogeneity) must be assessed before the procedure is initiated. When and only when the surgeon is satisfied that the laser is functioning appropriately should the treatment begin.

THE PROCEDURE

Having prepared the laser, the only thing missing is you.

The Patient Arrives

You are brought into the laser suite and seated on a reclining bed or a dentist-style chair. Depending on the centre's policy, a friend or family member may be permitted to accompany you.

The selected eye is confirmed and your other eye is covered with a protective shield. Both eyes should remain open throughout the procedure to prevent squeezing. (When you shut your eyes, the eyeballs themselves have a tendency to roll up, as if you were looking at your forehead.) More freezing drops are instilled to ensure that you will experience no pain. Remember that once an eye is anaesthetized, it has lost its protective sensation of pain. In order to prevent injury, and also to preserve the vital antiseptic environment, your hands should remain by your side. If your surgeon feels that it is necessary, you may be given a sedative. If you're too sleepy, your eyes may drift. Therefore, sedation is usually best avoided in PRK.

Your surgeon then lifts a contraption which bears striking resemblance to a medieval torture device. This *lid speculum* is designed to spread your eyelids, thereby exposing your cornea. Despite its ominous appearance, it is usually inserted without discomfort. You are asked to focus on a pinpoint light so that your visual axis can be identified. Once your eye is centered and the treatment zone is marked, the procedure begins for real.

Removal of the epithelium

PRK procedures require the removal of the front layer of the cornea, the *epithelium*. There are several options.

Mechanical	Removal of the epithelial layer with a scalpel, spatula, or brush.
Chemical	Removal of the epithelium after the application of alcohol.
Laser	The laser itself may be used to remove the epithelium.

Each technique has its advantages and disadvantages. The decision is probably best based on your surgeon's preference. Accuracy and speed are important, and the contribution of this preliminary step to the final outcome should not be underestimated.

The Laser

Finally. After months of agonizing anticipation, the moment has finally arrived. It is time to bring on the laser. The last thing anybody wants is for you to jump out of the chair as soon as you hear the laser for the first time. Therefore, in order to familiarize you with the sound, your surgeon will test-

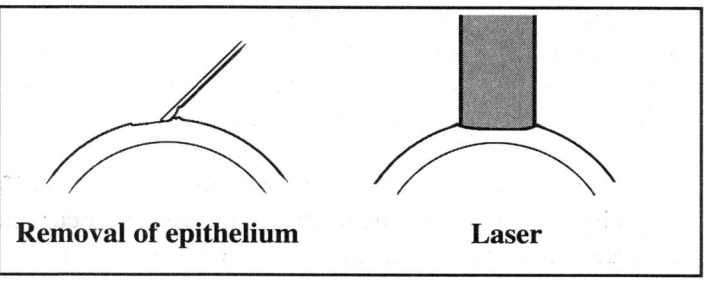

Removal of epithelium   **Laser**

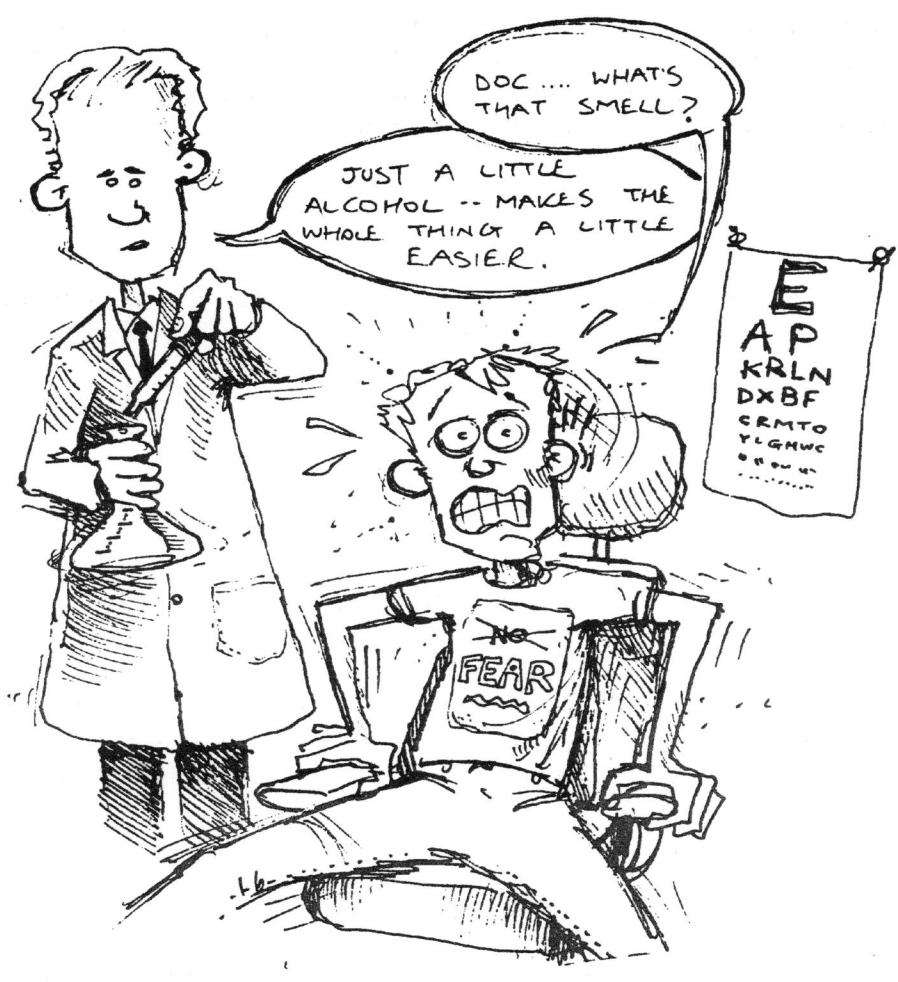

fire the laser. When both of you are ready, under microscopic visualization, your surgeon ensures that your eye is centred. Using a foot pedal control, the laser treatment is started. Depending on your refractive error, the actual laser time is anywhere from 10 to 40 seconds, but that's like saying a football game lasts 60 minutes. Stoppages in play must be taken into account. When your surgeon lifts his or her foot off the pedal, the laser stops. This is usually done when your surgeon detects eye decentration. Your eye may have drifted away from the target light. Interrupting the treatment allows you focus once again. When your surgeon is satisfied that your eye is properly centred, the foot goes down and the laser picks up where it left off. Many surgeons have an assistant call out the time remaining, and when you hear zero, it's all over.

The laser application itself lasts from a few seconds to over a minute, depending on the degree of correction required. The entire procedure, from sitting down to sitting up, usually takes less then ten minutes.

Eye Drops

The following compilation includes an incomplete listing of drugs (* denotes registered trade mark or trade name).

Steroids
> **Examples:** AK-Dex*, Econopred*, Flarex*, FML*, Inflamase*, Isolone Forte*, Maxidex*, Predforte*

> **Function:** Useful in preventing regression, inflammation, and NSAID-related corneal infiltrates

> **Disadvantages:** May cause increased IOP, cataract with prolonged use

Antibiotics
> **Examples:** Chloromycetin*, Ciloxan*, Garamycin*, Ilotycin*, Neosporin*, Ocuflox*, Polysporin*, Polytrim*, Sodium Sulamyd*, Tobrex*

> **Function:** Useful in preventing infection in immediate post operative period

> **Disadvantages:** Some antibiotics may delay epithelial healing

Steroid and Antibiotic Combinations
> **Examples:** Blephamide*, Cortisporin*, Dexacidin*, Maxitrol*, Poly-Pred*, Sulfacort*, TobraDex*

> **Function:** A convenient way of instilling two drugs in one drop

> **Disadvantages:** Unable to vary the dosage of each drug separately

Non-Steroidal Anti-Inflammatory Drugs (NSAID's)
<u>Examples</u>: Acular*, Indocid*, Ocufen*, Profenal*, Voltaren*

<u>Function</u>: Useful in preventing post-operative pain and inflammation

<u>Disadvantages</u>: May cause corneal infiltrates if used without steroids

Artificial Tears
<u>Examples</u>: Aquasite*, Cellufresh*, Hypotears*, Refresh*, Teargen II*, Tearisol*, Tears Naturale II*, Tears Plus*

<u>Function</u>: Useful in lubricating the post-operative eye, relieving irritation

<u>Disadvantages</u>: Tears with preservatives may cause corneal irritation, especially if used for prolonged periods

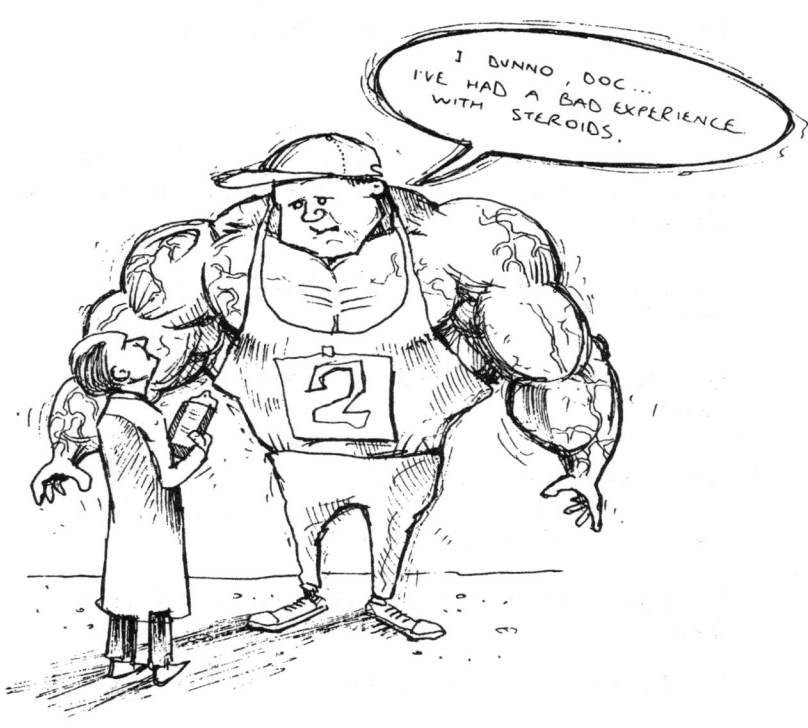

Using Eye Drops

1. Wash your hands before instilling any drops.

2. One drop per application is all you need for medicated drops.

3. Allow 3 to 5 minutes between different drops to allow proper absorption.

4. Shake the bottle before using it.

5. Tilt your head back, raise your eyelid, and squeeze the bottle gently.

6. Alternatively, you can create a small cup by pressing together the sides of your lower eyelid.

7. Avoid touching your eyes and eyelashes with the bottle tip (to prevent contamination).

POST-OP

The first minute

Before you start jumping up and down in celebration, certain things must be done. Drops are placed in the eye to jumpstart the healing process. A steroid, a NSAID, and an antibiotic are frequently the drops of choice. In addition, a bandage contact lens may be placed on the cornea. When you sit up, things are blurry. This is normal and to be expected. The eye feels comfortable, however, because the effect of the anaesthetic eye drops lingers. After last minute instructions from the laser suite staff, you are set free.

The first hour

Things get worse before they get better. When the effect of the anaesthesia wears off, the eye becomes sensitive. Sometimes even painful. It is difficult to predict. With the use of a bandage contact lens and NSAID eye drops, the incidence and severity of pain is much less than it used to be. Furthermore, adding insult to injury, your vision remains poor. With the possibility of pain and decreased vision, you may not feel like going back to work. It is a good idea to have someone take you home.

The first day

The first twenty-four hours are the worst. Discomfort or pain may develop in the first few hours and may persist for the rest of the day. This, in conjunction with blurred vision, makes you feel a little under the weather. There are people who view a four limb amputation as just a flesh wound, and they are not slowed down in the least by a measly PRK procedure. Most mortals instead prefer to spend the first day at home, ideally being waited on, hand and foot, by a sympathetic friend or family member. Eye drops should be used as prescribed and painkillers may be taken for severe pain. You are usually seen on the first or second day after surgery in order to ensure that the healing process is underway.

The first week

The second day, you feel better. The pain is diminished, and it is unlikely that you require painkillers. Vision remains poor, and may, in fact, be a little worse as the contact lens becomes coated with protein. If you had the procedure in one eye, you may find yourself wanting to return to work, even though your depth perception may be impaired. Your job requirements should be taken into account, however, as operating heavy machinery or playing Wimbledon may not be wise. Generally, it is inadvisable to return to work before the epithelium has healed, because of the risk of infection. If you had bilateral surgery performed, forget work and tennis entirely for the first few days. It might be a good time to work on the karaoke skills.

The first week is critical. Most sight-threatening complications, if they're going to happen, occur during this time. Consequently, the eye drops should be used as if your sight depended on it and your follow-up appointments should be not be missed. In general, you should be seen on a regular basis until the epithelium has completely healed. Typically, this should take about three days, but that's also what the post-office says. Be prepared for some variability, but at the very least there should be a daily reduction in the size of the epithelial defect. Specifically, patients over forty years of age may endure a prolonged healing period. Vision also improves during this first week, most dramatically when the contact lens is removed. You are usually seen around the one week mark to ensure that things are healing satisfactorily. At this stage, your uncorrected vision may be recorded around the 20/60 level, give or take depending on your pre-operative refractive error.

The first month

Vision gradually improves. Unless you had a high degree of pre-operative myopia, 20/40 uncorrected vision should be achieved sometime during the first month, often in the first two weeks. Best corrected vision may be reduced early in this time period, however it usually returns to pre-operative levels by the end of the first month. If your eye has been overcorrected, as is often the plan, you may have to use the accommodative power of your crystalline lens to compensate for this new hyperopia. This happens naturally, and is not usually a problem unless you are over the age of forty. In that case, your accommodative reserve is likely low and eye-strain symptoms may result. A follow-up appointment at this time is the basis of certain decisions. By now your doctor has an idea how your cornea is responding.

Regression

Now would be a good time to learn a little bit about this issue, because it comes into play in the first month. PRK would be so much simpler without a phenomenon known as *myopic regression*. As the cornea heals following PRK, the refractive error tends to drift back toward myopia. It is a proven, predictable, treatable event but it makes everything a little more complicated.

For those who truly believe that everything in life is metaphored on a golf course, regression is a putt. A downhill putt with a severe right to left break. The hole is straight ahead, but if you aim directly at it, you'll miss it to the left. In order to sink the putt, you have to aim away from the hole and let it roll back.

In PRK, you have to aim high. If you aim for a one month post-operative refraction of plano (zero) and 20/20 uncorrected vision, things will be great for the short term. As time goes by and regression takes over, the final refraction one year down the road will be disappointingly myopic. That's why your surgeon usually aims to overcorrect and leave you slightly farsighted soon after surgery. Predictable regression will bring a one month grumbling hyperope to a six month smiling emmetrope.

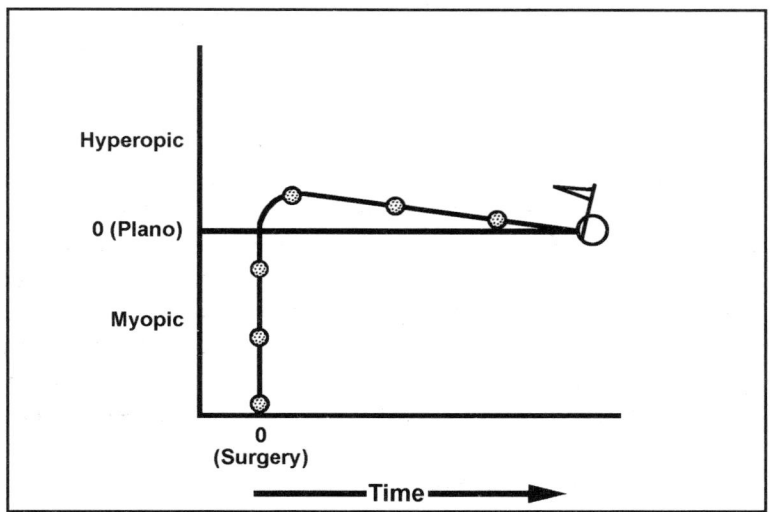

Professional golfers think in terms of a two-putt. From anywhere on the green, they feel they should be able to get the ball in the hole in two strokes. If you're three feet away, they would like to sink it in one shot, but from twelve feet, two putts is pretty good. Now imagine that one foot equals one Diopter. A decent surgeon should be able to get a 3 D myope to 20/20 in one attempt. Not all of the time, mind you; even Fred Couples misses a few of those, but most of the time.

A 12 D myope is a different story. Now you have to think in terms of two shots. Your surgeon would, of course, like to do it in one. Still, it may be worth planning for two.

Any golfer knows that downhill putts are tricky. It is much easier to gauge distance and direction when putting uphill. For this reason, if you're going to miss a putt, it is better to leave yourself an easy uphill putt to save par.

Similarly, it is much easier to achieve surgical success from the myopic side of emmetropia. If you started at -12 D and find yourself -3 D post-PRK, you're in good shape. You're just a short uphill putt from plano. If, however, your first PRK leaves you a +3 D hyperope, you're in a tricky situation. That second putt is not a gimme.

For these reasons, deciding on PRK goals is not straightforward. Your surgeon would like to aim for a slight overcorrection, thereby allowing regression to work its charm. If the overcorrection is too great, however, you may end up in a difficult farsighted position. Overall, it is a tricky balance and your surgeon must take all of these issues into consideration.

As if things weren't complicated enough, there are two more factors which enter into the equation. Continuing with our golf analogy, the player must know his or her putter inside and out. The golfer must know that if he or she hits a putt with a six inch backswing, the ball will travel forty inches on flat ground. Every golf club is unique and it is only from practice that these predictable tendencies are discovered. The same applies to lasers.

In golf, once you've hit your putt, its out of your hands. Sure you can lean your body hard to the left or to the right, but there is no scientific evidence that you're doing anything but making a fool of yourself. Now if only you could run beside the ball with a battery-powered fan. If you want the ball to break more, you turn up the power on the fan. If it looks like the ball is breaking too much, you turn down the power.

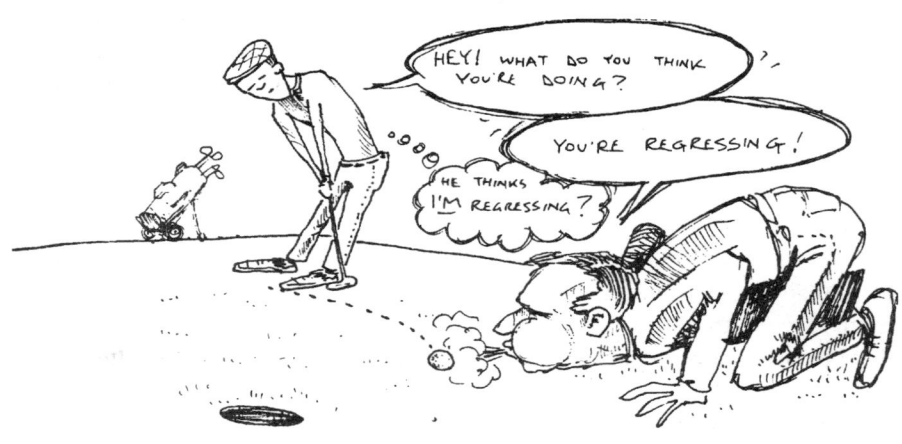

Eye drops are the fan. Steroid drops may inhibit regression. Therefore, if your eye is myopic or plano immediately post-operatively, steroids may be used aggressively to try and prevent regression. In contrast, if your eye is too hyperopic in the early post-operative period, steroids may be withdrawn to encourage regression.

Recent studies have attempted to identify predisposing elements in the hope of preventing the problem from developing. The following factors may increase your risk of significant regression.

- Regression after PRK in the first eye
- Higher pre-operative refractive error
- Smaller treatment zones
- Oral contraceptive use
- Sun exposure post-operatively

It is important to realize that myopic regression must be understood, predicted, prevented, compensated for, and treated.

The first month continued

Returning to the post-operative course, at the one month stage: If your eye is undercorrected (still myopic), there is a good chance that you will require PRK enhancement. If you have been using drops, your doctor may recommend tapering off the drops quickly which will allow your refraction to stabilize. The sooner you're off the steroids, the sooner the eye stabilizes and the sooner retreatment can be performed. It is usually advisable to wait three to six months after surgery in order to ensure that your refraction is stable. In some cases, *monovision* (see Chapter 4) may be a reasonable alternative to retreatment.

If your eye is perfectly corrected at one month, that is a refraction of plano (zero), your happiness may be short-lived. Although you may still end up with a good result, regression is working against you. Continued frequent use of topical steroids may prevent your prescription from drifting toward the minus side. Although retreatment may be avoided, you should be prepared for that possibility down the road. Monovision may be an acceptable alternative.

If your eye is slightly over-corrected, chances are things are perfectly on schedule. If you have been using eye drops, your doctor may instruct you to reduce their frequency, perhaps from four times a day to three times a day. Expected regression over the next few months should drop you in for a soft landing around plano.

If your eye is greatly over-corrected, regression becomes your friend. Instead of preventing with eye drops, regression should be encouraged. For this reason, your doctor may suggest stopping or rapidly tapering off the drops. Once the refraction has dropped into the desired range, the steroid drops can be restarted.

The first year

It takes a few months for the eye to stabilize. The refractive error may gradually drift back toward myopia. Uncorrected vision is usually improving, however glare symptoms may present night time difficulties early on. The eye may feel a little irritated from time to time, especially the first thing in the morning. You may continue to take eye drops for a few months, but the dosage usually decreases as time goes by. Follow-up appointments are monthly at first, and thereafter depend on your progress. If all goes well, by six months, you are stable at plano, your uncorrected vision is excellent, and those night time symptoms are a thing of the past.

RESULTS

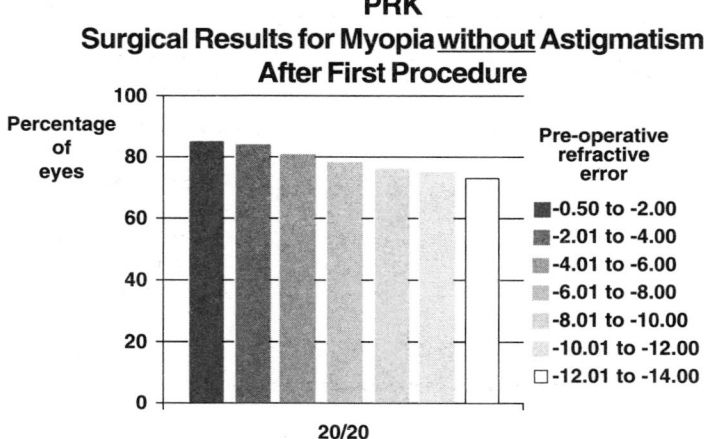

PRK
Surgical Results for Myopia without Astigmatism
After First Procedure

Percentage of eyes

Pre-operative refractive error

■ -0.50 to -2.00
■ -2.01 to -4.00
▒ -4.01 to -6.00
▒ -6.01 to -8.00
▒ -8.01 to -10.00
░ -10.01 to -12.00
☐ -12.01 to -14.00

20/20

Post-operative uncorrected visual acuity

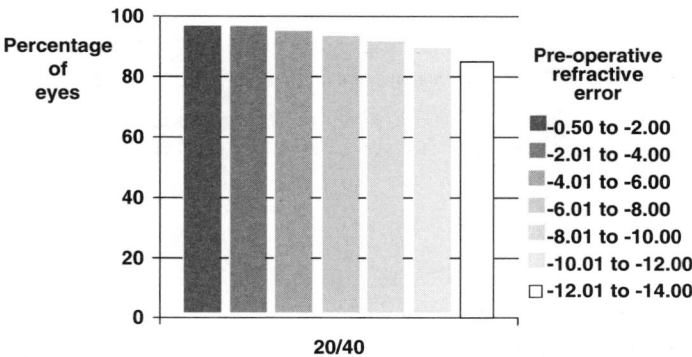

PRK
Surgical Results for Myopia without Astigmatism
After First Procedure

Post-operative uncorrected visual acuity

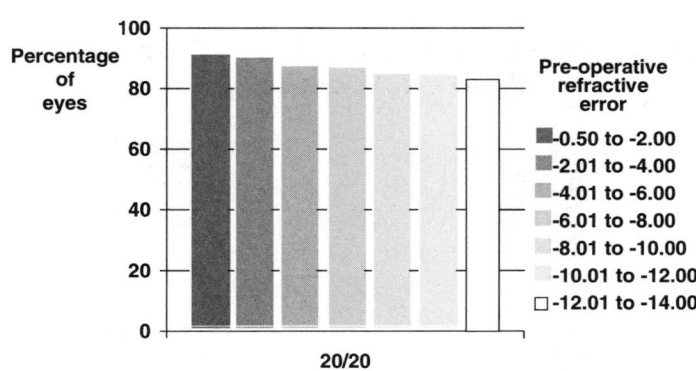

PRK
Surgical Results for Myopia without Astigmatism
After All Procedures

Post-operative uncorrected visual acuity

PRK
Surgical Results for Myopia <u>without</u> Astigmatism
After All Procedures

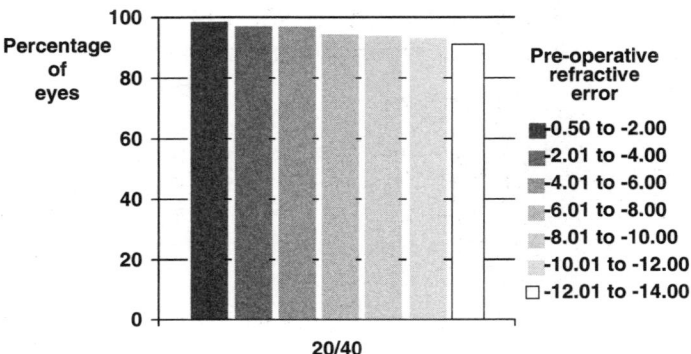

Post-operative uncorrected visual acuity

PRK
Surgical Results for Myopia <u>without</u> Astigmatism
Within ± 1.00 D of Intended Correction
After First Procedure

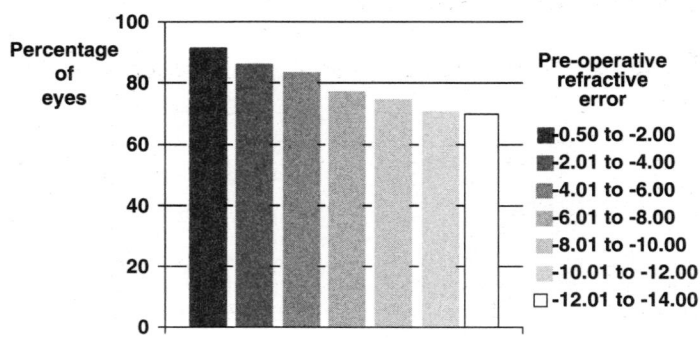

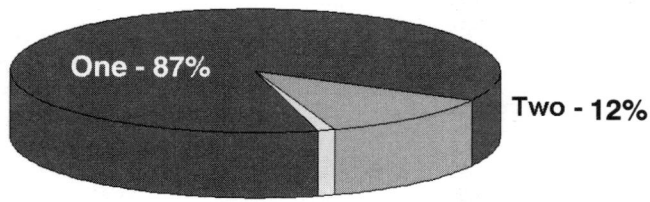

**PRK
Surgical Results for Myopia
Number of Treatments per Eye**

One - 87%

Two - 12%

Three or more - 1 %

COMPLICATIONS

Undercorrection

If the refractive error is still myopic after the surgery, the terms *undercorrection* or *under response* are used.

Why?: In the perfect surgical world which everyone is seeking, all patients are plano post-operatively. Because of individual variation in wound healing, imperfect surgical algorithms, and factors which we have not yet appreciated, this is not a 100% predictable procedure.

Numbers: The percentage of people who require retreatment for myopia depends on the degree of pre-operative refractive error. For myopes in the mild to moderate range, this number is around 10%. In addition, the retreatment rate depends upon doctor and patient satisfaction and confidence, and on the philosophy of retreatment for small residual refractive errors. Some people who have a post-operative visual acuity of 20/25 may undergo retreatment if they are dissatisfied and their surgeon believes that the second or third operation offers a reasonable risk/benefit ratio.

Treatment: The treatment depends on the extent of undercorrection, the degree of patient satisfaction (or dissatisfaction), the confidence/aggressiveness of the surgeon, and the time course. In general, the options are to do something or to do nothing. "Something" usually means retreatment.

Also known as PRK enhancement or touch-up, there is no point in sugar-coating the issue. It is a second (or third or fourth) procedure. The first one didn't achieve perfect results, so it is time to try again. There's nothing wrong with that. Remember, two putts is par for the course, and there are people who have had four or five procedures who end up with an excellent result.

If? Conservative is not a four letter word. It is better to avoid a second procedure if possible. Every time you go under the laser, the same risks present themselves all over again. If you end up having a million PRK procedures, those one in a million risks suddenly become a bit of a factor. So rather than tempting fate, it is usually better to attempt conservative treatment first. If it works, great. You've avoided unnecessary surgery. If it doesn't work, what have you lost? You can then have the retreatment knowing that at least you tried the other, less risky, alternatives.

A second procedure should not be attempted without a clearly identified problem and a specific goal. You shouldn't draw in blackjack when you're sitting at 20, and you shouldn't go looking for trouble trying to vault from almost perfect to absolutely perfect. In general, you should think twice about retreatment if your uncorrected vision is 20/40 or better. If you can see well enough to drive without glasses, why rock the boat? As always, there are exceptions.

When? The key is stability. You wouldn't try to putt the ball while its still rolling. That would make the shot infinitely more difficult and less predictable. When your cornea has healed to the point where it is not changing any more, then, and only then, should retreatment be performed. Usually, this means about

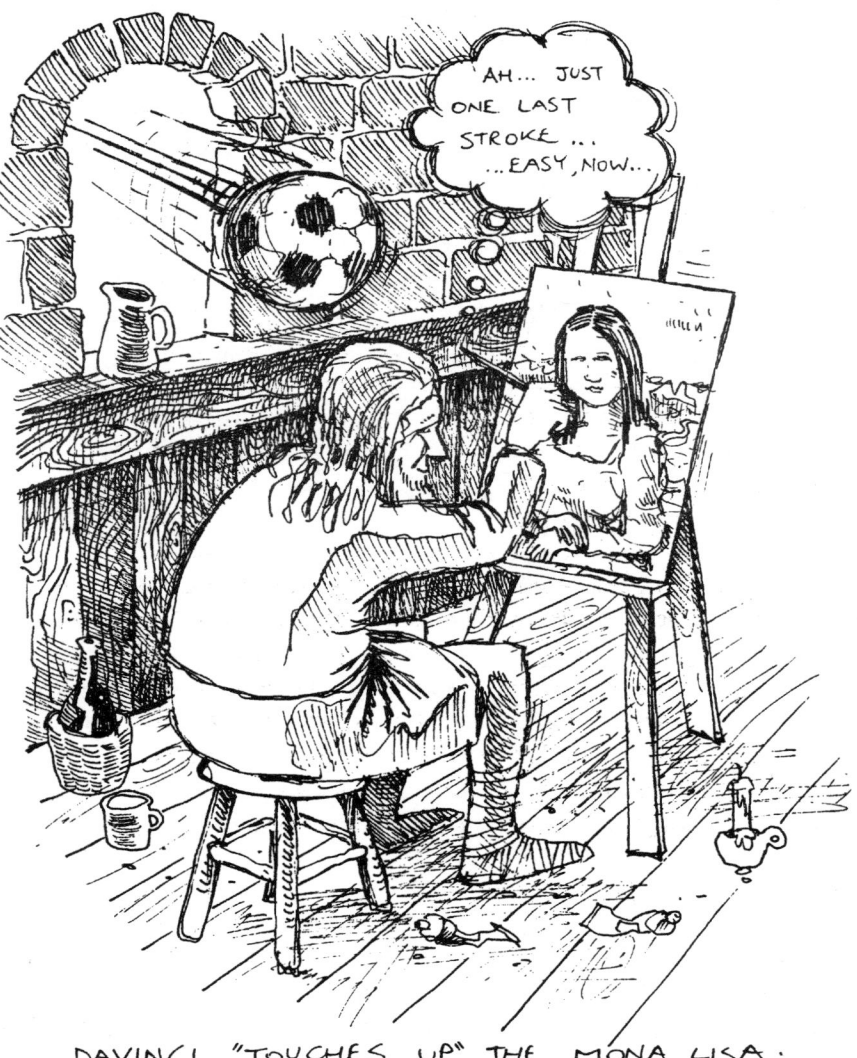

DAVINCI "TOUCHES UP" THE MONA LISA.

three to six months after surgery, but the actual time can vary in either direction.

How? The post-PRK eye is not the same as a virgin cornea. It is different (anatomy), it behaves differently (physiology), and it should be treated differently (surgically). Although the details are not important, one principle is worth noting. The nature and extent of the surgery are directly related to the reason for retreatment in the first place. That is, an eye with a mild undercorrection is treated differently than an eye suffering primarily from glare.

The second surgery does not have to be the same procedure as the first.

PRK after PRK: This alternative probably makes the most sense. Unless there were complications of the initial procedure that suggest otherwise, probably the reasons that led you to PRK in the first place will lead you back.

LASIK after PRK: If there were difficulties related to epithelial healing after the first procedure, retreatment with LASIK may prevent a recurrence of the problem.

RK after PRK: Although it is theoretically possible to perform the procedures in this order, the recent trend is the reverse. It is a bit of a scientific paradox to give up CD's for LP's.

Prognosis: Undercorrected eyes usually respond well to retreatment and have an excellent visual prognosis.

Overcorrection

If the post-operative refractive error is hyperopic, the eye has over responded and is termed *overcorrected.*

Why? Once again, the same factors which contribute to undercorrection or under response come into play. People over the age of forty seem to be slightly predisposed to developing an overcorrection. The reasons for this are being investigated. In addition, overcorrection is seen more frequently when greater degrees of myopia are treated.

Numbers: Because of the conservative treatment algorithms which are usually employed, significant overcorrection is uncommon and decreasing in frequency.

Treatment: The treatment is dependent on the extent of overcorrection and the age of the patient. Young people with significant hyperopia can use their crystalline lens to compensate for their new refractive error. Presbyopes, conversely, are unable to accommodate at all, and the slightest degree of hyperopia can be a problem.

The most important element of overcorrection is avoidance. Those downhill putts are tricky, and it is far better to be undercorrected than overcorrected.

Stimulation of regression is the goal for hyperopia in the immediate post-operative period. Discontinuation of steroids, initiation of other eye drops, extended wear contact lens use, and corneal scraping have all been advocated. Should the eye remain hyperopic, glasses and contacts are, of course, options. However, surgical intervention may be considered and warranted. The specific modalities of treatment are the same as for primary hyperopia (See Chapter 10)

Prognosis: The use of a laser to retreat small overcorrections is often successful.

Pain

For many people, this is a big deterrent when considering PRK. It takes tremendous will power to pick up the telephone voluntarily and ask to be put in pain.

Why? As anybody who has had a fingernail in the eye will tell you, a corneal abrasion is painful. That situation is not very different from PRK. The epithelium is removed, leaving a raw, sensitive surface. Until the epithelial layer regenerates, the eye may be painful.

Numbers: Most people who have PRK experience some

discomfort. With new techniques, severe pain is reported in less than 10% of patients. Studies demonstrate that pain begins, on average, one hour after the surgery and becomes maximal about eight hours after the procedure. Furthermore, pain decreases to acceptable levels around the twenty-four hour mark. In general, once you endure the first day, the worst is behind you. With current treatment, many people have no pain, only irritation.

Treatment: Patching may be used to protect the eye from irritation. It not only reduces pain, but also promotes epithelial healing. Vision is obstructed, however, which is annoying in unilateral surgery and intolerable in bilateral cases.

A bandage contact lens also reduces pain by protecting the raw corneal surface. There is, unfortunately, a very slight associated risk of infection, as a foreign material has now been introduced into the eye.

Pills (eg. codeine) are often helpful for short-term pain control, but have significant side effects.

Non-Steroidal Anti-Inflammatory Drugs (NSAID) eye drops are gaining popularity, but some studies suggest that they may slow epithelial healing.

Topical anaesthetic eye drops have traditionally been regarded as dangerous, but are currently under investigation.

The use of these treatment modalities varies from centre to centre, but a trend is emerging. Many surgeons are now recommending the use of a bandage contact lens in conjunction with NSAID eye drops, plus oral medication if necessary. This combination has been demonstrated to prevent or relieve post-operative pain in the majority of patients. It is worth observing that a small minority of patients complain of pain regardless of the treatment program.

Delayed Epithelial Healing

Post-operatively, the area of epithelial defect gets smaller and smaller on a daily basis. In the majority of people, the epithelium is completely healed by three days. In a small minority, however, there is a prolonged period of healing.

In many contests, it is better to be the tortoise than the hare. When it comes to epithelial healing, conversely, the rabbit has the right idea. Delayed healing can contribute to the development of further problems.

> Why? Often there is no apparent reason, however contributing factors may sometimes be identified. A poorly fit bandage contact lens may be the problem. In addition, toxicity from eye drops may affect epithelial healing. General health problems such as diabetes may also be a factor.
>
> Numbers: This is an infrequent complication, seen in approximately 0.2% of cases.
>
> Treatment: If a specific problem is identified, it should be addressed. The prescribed medications, particularly steroids and NSAIDs, should be reassessed and possibly reduced or discontinued. Consideration should be given to removing the contact lens and either replacing it, or patching the eye until epithelialization has occurred.
>
> Prognosis: Even eyes with delayed epithelialization usually heal completely. They just take their time. Prolonged healing, however, may be associated with an increased risk of corneal infection and haze.

Haze/scarring

One of the most common post-operative problems is the development of corneal haze. Usually at the level of the anterior stroma, this haze may vary in degree. There are scales which attempt to quantify the extent of haze, however the details are of secondary importance. The haze can be anywhere along the spectrum from barely discernable to severe. Corneal scarring is at the far end of the spectrum and is distinguished from haze by its irreversibility and visual significance. Vision may not be affected by haze alone. In fact, many people who have significant haze will not even be aware of it. Others complain of "starbursts". Typically, this is a night time effect where lights do not appear distinct.

Why? Haze and scarring are not always predictable, however certain factors place an eye at increased risk, including:

- Delayed epithelial healing
- Small treatment zones
- Greater treatment depth
- High myopia pre-operatively

Numbers: Haze is generally an early phenomenon. Studies demonstrate that it begins at a few weeks, peaks at approximately three months post-operatively, and gradually decreases over the following two years. Although it is not uncommon to encounter visually significant haze in the first few months, (7%), by the one year mark, that number drops to about 2%. Newer laser delivery systems and protocols continue to reduce the incidence of haze.

Treatment: Patience is the best early treatment. In most cases, time will cure the haze and eliminate the starbursts. A number of different treatment modalities have been proposed for persistent haze, including topical steroids, topical NSAIDs, and retreatment with laser if myopic regression is an associated factor.

Prognosis: Haze usually improves to the extent that it is not a significant problem. Scarring tends to persist and an unfortunate few are left with reduced best-corrected visual acuity and residual night time difficulties despite retreatments. Scarring does tend to clear gradually over two to three years. If PRK retreatment and time does not resolve the problem, there are other surgical procedures available, such as lamellar corneal grafts.

Halos

Also seen at night, halos are entirely different than sunbursts. As the name suggests, halos are often described as a concentric circle surrounding a light.

Why? It is becoming increasingly apparent that halos are the result of a size mismatch. In an ideal situation, the pupil is the same size or smaller than the zone of laser treatment. This means that all of the light which reaches the retina has gone through the treated part of the cornea. In daylight, in most eyes, this is the case. In darkness, however, the pupils dilate. If the pupil now becomes larger than the zone of laser treatment, light can then enter the eye without going through the treated part of the cornea. Halos result. Prolonged use of steroid drops has been observed to cause temporary pupillary dilatation which may exacerbate this effect.

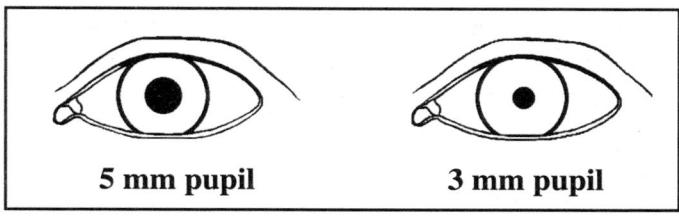

5 mm pupil   **3 mm pupil**

Numbers: The chance of developing halos is directly related to the size of the treatment zone. Early studies, using a 4 mm zone, demonstrated an overwhelming 75% incidence of halos. When larger zones were used, this number dropped. A 5 mm zone gave a 40% to 50% incidence of halos, and at 6 mm, the incidence drops to single digits. New studies using a 7 mm treatment zone estimate the incidence of halos to be in the 1% to 2% range.

Treatment: Armed with this knowledge, the best idea is to prevent halos using a large treatment zone. Newer techniques of laser programming suggest that these larger zones may be treated in a safe manner. If bothersome halos do present themselves, most times they are related to early healing effects, and improve spontaneously. Patience is, once again, the best answer. For incapacitating persistent halos, retreatment with larger zones may be helpful, providing that the depth of treatment limits are not exceeded.

<u>Prognosis:</u> With newer techniques, patience, and treatment, it is uncommon for halos to become a significant problem. Also working to your advantage is the fact that pupils tend to become smaller with age.

Corneal ulcer

Whether it is in your stomach or in your eye, it is never a good idea to get an ulcer. A corneal ulcer is an infection and it is one of the most feared complications of PRK. Because it may develop in the central part of the cornea, the area where the protective epithelium was removed, it is potentially vision threatening.

<u>Why?</u> If there were specific reasons why this happens, then it would be predictable and therefore, preventable. Unfortunately, this is not the case. Like apartment hunters in Manhattan, there are bacteria everywhere just looking for a cozy environment to call home. Despite meticulous pre-operative, intra-operative, and post-operative care, sometimes an infection can develop for no apparent reason. The important thing is to reduce the risk by strictly adhering to pre-operative and post-operative instructions. Antibiotic eye drops and follow-up appointments are strategic preventative measures that should not be ignored. Lifestyle choices that promote a healthy immune system are also protective.

<u>Numbers:</u> Significant corneal ulcers occur in approximately 0.1% (one in a thousand) cases.

<u>Treatment:</u> If you are unfortunate enough to develop a corneal ulcer, your prognosis is much better if it is detected and managed sooner rather than later. Treatment includes removing the bandage contact lens, sending it off to the laboratory for culture along with a sample from your eye, and the prescription of frequent antibiotic eye drops.

Prognosis: The prognosis is variable, depending on the location, severity, and time elapsed before treatment. When the ulcer heals, a central corneal scar may be left. Therefore, the threat of visual loss should not be ignored.

Irregular astigmatism

The smooth, regular surface of the cornea may become irregular following PRK.

Why? Poor fixation or eye centering, in addition to the post-operative healing process, may cause irregularities in the contour.

Numbers: Significant irregular astigmatism may be seen in 0.3% of post-operative eyes.

Treatment: The management of irregular astigmatism, in contrast to regular astigmatism, is difficult. Wearing glasses or soft contact lenses does not correct this problem, as the astigmatism varies throughout the cornea. Likewise, surgical treatment is difficult. If significant visual loss occurs, a rigid contact lens may be useful, because it becomes a new smooth refracting surface of the cornea.

Prognosis: Irregular astigmatism is responsible for a considerable fraction of the eyes which lose "best-corrected" visual acuity.

Increased intraocular pressure (IOP)

If the IOP becomes elevated, post-operatively, optic nerve damage can ensue. When this happens, vision may be threatened and the term glaucoma is used.

Why? PRK does not, in itself, cause the IOP to increase. The culprit is usually the steroid eye drops which are prescribed post-operatively. It is well established that prolonged use of these medications may cause elevated IOP. Not surprisingly, this phenomenon has been observed following refractive surgery.

Numbers: The frequency and degree of increased IOP is extremely variable. Depending on the study, elevated IOP has been demonstrated in anywhere from 1% to 25% of post-PRK patients. The most likely reason for this variability is that many things can affect IOP, including the duration, frequency, dosage, and type of topical steroid prescribed. Genetic predisposition is also a factor.

Treatment: With judicious use of low potency steroids and a tapering regimen, elevations of IOP may be prevented. If it does occur, the increased IOP usually responds well to either stopping the steroid and/or adding another pressure-reducing eye drop.

Prognosis: Increased IOP is usually not a problem in itself. It only becomes a problem if ocular damage results. Although there have been reports of some visual loss from increased IOP following refractive surgery, this happens only rarely. Because visual loss, when it happens, is irreversible, prevention is the key. Regular follow-up appointments are essential, and adjustments to the eye drop regimen should be made only by your doctor.

Cataract

The prolonged post-operative use of steroid eye drops has been reported to cause cataracts.

Why? This is a complication of prolonged topical steroid use, which has been observed in many diseases where such long term treatment is necessary. In the case of refractive surgery, it is like adding insult to injury. You have PRK to improve your vision only to develop a cataract which interferes with your vision.

Numbers: Fortunately, cataracts are rare (0.1%) in the context of refractive surgery. By prescribing less potent steroids and by tapering the dosage, cataracts are becoming more and more just a theoretical complication.

<u>Treatment:</u> If a cataract does develop, it is irreversible. When it is visually significant, a cataract extraction (see Chapter 8) is advisable. Prevention and early recognition, as always, are paramount.

<u>Prognosis:</u> Even if a significant cataract does develop, modern surgical techniques will still provide very good vision in the vast majority of patients.

Decentration

Imagine a donut with the hole a little off to one side. Decentration is what happens when the treatment zone is not exactly in the right position. The resulting effect depends on the degree of decentration. Fortunately the eye is quite forgiving in this regard and if the decentration is small, there will likely be no noticeable effect. Larger discrepancies may result in blurred vision, halos, night glare, and possibly even double vision.

<u>Why?</u> Centration of the laser during treatment is the responsibility of both the doctor and the patient. The patient must concentrate on keeping their gaze fixed on the target. The surgeon should watch for any drift from this position, and interrupt treatment when necessary. It is a natural reaction to push your chin down into your chest, as if trying to escape from the laser. This instinct should be fought, because it can cause decentration. Keeping the eye properly positioned is not always as easy as it sounds, for either party, and for this reason, some new laser machines have incorporated eye-tracking sensors into their hardware.

<u>Numbers:</u> The risk of significant decentration is low, in the 2% to 4% range. As techniques improve, with larger treatment zones, improved surgeon awareness, and technological advances, this problem should continue to decrease in frequency.

<u>Treatment:</u> Prevention is the best form of treatment. Some

surgeons prefer to instill a pre-operative eye drop which constricts the pupil into a pinpoint. This, in theory, makes it easier to visualize eye decentration. This drop, however, is not without side effects. The constricted pupil, for example, may shift off centre. Treatment of visually significant decentration may employ the use of pupil-constricting eye drops or contact lenses, however PRK retreatment may be necessary.

Prognosis: With appropriate treatment, most symptoms of decentration improve or resolve.

Ptosis

A droopy eyelid is referred to as a ptosis.

Why? Ptosis is sometimes seen following any refractive surgery and has been attributed to the required use of a lid speculum intraoperatively. Also, topical steroids have been thought to play a role.

Numbers: The droop is usually mild, often barely noticable, and may vary throughout the day. It occurs uncommonly, perhaps in 1% of eyes.

Treatment: Patience and tapering the steroid eye drops usually does the trick.

Prognosis: In most people, given enough time, post-PRK ptosis improves and ultimately disappears. Persistent ptosis can be treated with further surgery.

Recurrent corneal erosion

Usually when someone receives a scratch to the eye, a corneal abrasion results. In most cases, everything heals up perfectly, as if it had never happened. Then suddenly, maybe months after the injury, this person might wake up in the morning to a sharp pain in the same eye. They see their doctor who informs them that the abrasion has returned. I was alone in bed, the patient protests. There was no fingernail for miles. The culprit is the recurrent corneal erosion syndrome, and it can be seen after PRK as well.

Why? Anytime the epithelium is removed from the cornea, the layer is forced to regenerate. Cells multiply and cover the area of defect. In a few unfortunate instances, this new layer is not as good as the old one. You may be minding your own business one day only to suddenly experience the same pain as you felt immediately after the injury or operation. The epithelium has come off and you're left with an abrasion.

Numbers: It is uncommon for recurrent corneal erosions to develop after PRK, on the order of 0.3% of operated eyes. When it happens, this condition is typically encountered the first thing in the morning and can occur even months after the procedure. The pain may be anywhere from mild to severe, and it usually resolves quickly and spontaneously.

Treatment: If your doctor observes an area of frank epithelial defect, an eye patch may be applied to encourage healing. Once the epithelium is intact, the goal of treatment is to prevent further recurrences. Eye drops which draw fluid from the cornea are often useful in promoting epithelial adherence. If the problem recurs despite these conservative measures, more aggressive treatment, such as further laser application, may be worthwhile.

Prognosis: It is rare for recurrent erosion syndrome to become a persistent significant problem.

PRK Summary

Advantages
- No risk of globe perforation
- Reduced risk of serious complications
- Predictable effect in low myopes
- Longer-term studies than LASIK
- FDA approved
- May be effective in myopia *and* hyperopia
- No significant structural weakness of cornea

Disadvantages
- Possible post-operative pain
- Possible long-term eye drops
- Visual improvement gradual
- Epithelium removed
- Myopic regression
- Less predictable in high myopes
- Haze

Best in...

Low myopia: The best results with the least complications are seen in patients with myopia less than 6 D. Coincidentally, that is close to the FDA limit for PRK.

Safety first: Less than twenty percent of the corneal thickness is removed during PRK. There is virtually no risk of intra-operative penetration into the eye, and the structural integrity of the cornea is largely intact post-operatively.

Americans: Until LASIK is approved by the FDA, it might be difficult to find an American surgeon willing to perform that procedure. PRK may be the only laser game in town.

Technophiliacs: Unless you spend your days watching black and white TV, wearing shoes without air in them, and putting saccharin in your coffee, you have demonstrated a certain faith in technology. For some, the precision and excitement of laser eye surgery may be irresistible, when compared with RK.

6

LASER IN SITU KERATOMILEUSIS (LASIK)

THE ROAD TO 1997

In 1949, an eye surgeon had a bright idea. If the problem with a myopic eye was that the cornea was too steep, then why not reshape it. Part of the cornea was excised and using a cryolathe, it was resculpted then reimplanted. This procedure, *Myopic Keratomileusis (MKM),* was the forerunner of current techniques.

Automated Lamellar Keratoplasty (ALK) was devised using the same premise of reshaping the cornea. The procedure is performed under topical anaesthesia using a machine called a *microkeratome.* This surgical

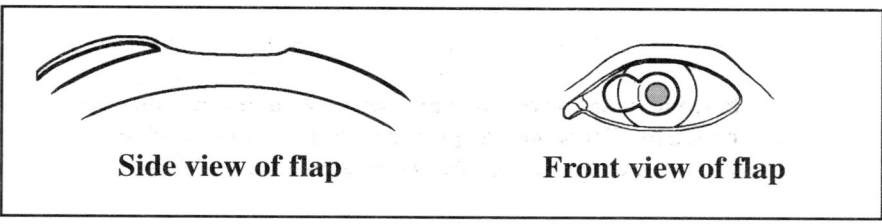

Side view of flap   **Front view of flap**

instrument is essentially an automatic knife which operates with extreme precision. It is capable of cutting very thin and accurate sections of tissue, and when applied to the cornea, a flap can be created.

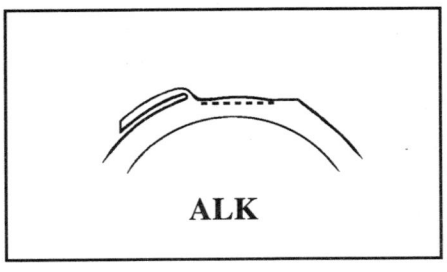

ALK

Once the flap is cut, it is flipped over to expose the underlying corneal stromal bed. This is known as the *first cut,* and is purely a preparatory move. Now is when the real surgery begins. In order to change the refractive power of the cornea, stromal tissue must be removed. ALK utilizes the microkeratome to make another sweep of the cornea, called the *refractive cut.* This time, instead of creating a flap of epithelium and stroma, the microkeratome actually cuts and removes a smaller disc of stromal tissue. The flap is then flipped back into its original position and the surgery is complete. The resulting cornea is missing a slice of tissue which confers a change in refraction.

Laser In Situ Keratomileusis (LASIK) is a procedure which combines the principles of ALK with the precision and glamour of PRK. Just as in ALK, a microkeratome performs the access cut and a corneal flap is created. Instead of excising corneal tissue mechanically, however, the stroma is thinned using the excimer laser. The desired refractive change is programmed into the laser, which in turn works its magic on the exposed stromal bed. When the laser has finished, the flap is repositioned, and a refractive change has been accomplished.

With its more precise centering, more precise ablation, and lenticular ablation instead of parallel excision, LASIK has several advantages over ALK. Although myopic ALK is currently being performed, it appears to be destined for extinction as hordes of ophthalmologists abandon this procedure for the greener pastures of LASIK.

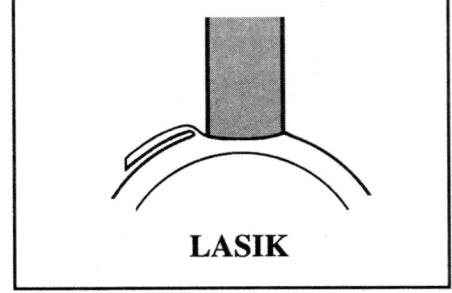

LASIK

Is LASIK For You?

Anybody can drive a car. And if you can drive a Cadillac, you can drive a Miata. Still, although both may be fine vehicles, certain people are better suited to each car. A family of six with a group discount at the Hair Club for Men may not be ideal owners of a Miata. The same principle applies to LASIK. Unless there are specific reasons otherwise, this procedure can theoretically be performed on anybody.

Unlike PRK, LASIK has not yet been approved by the FDA. Criteria for LASIK candidates, therefore, have not been firmly established. Without the benefit of FDA guidelines, the question which has yet to be answered conclusively is, for whom is LASIK best suited. The added problem, as described earlier, relates to the FDA belief that LASIK is an "off-label" use of the excimer laser. Until the issue is resolved once and for all, the ability of American patients and surgeons to choose LASIK may be somewhat impeded.

Contraindications

LASIK should not be performed, or performed with caution, in people who have certain *contraindications:*

> Mental Health - LASIK should be avoided in patients if they or their legal guardians are unable to understand fully the risks and benefits of the procedure.

> General Health - In contrast to PRK, where epithelial healing plays an important role in the success of surgery, LASIK has no such requirement. Consequently, individuals who are not PRK candidates because of general medical concerns may be at less risk with LASIK. Still, such surgery should be entered into with caution and awareness.

> Pregnancy/Nursing

> Ocular disease - LASIK may not be advisable in patients with significant ocular disease and, specifically, the following:

>> *One functional eye* - If the best-corrected vision in one eye is worse than 20/40, the procedure may not

be justified considering the risk/benefit ratio. Operating on the one good eye is just too risky, whereas it is not worth treating the bad eye because of limited potential benefit.

Corneal disease - (eg. keratoconus, severe dry eye, herpes simplex/zoster keratitis)

Unstable refractive error

Previous eye surgery - The success of LASIK may be compromised by previous eye surgery.

PREPARING FOR LASIK

Preparing the patient and the laser

The preparation for LASIK is similar to that for PRK.

Preparing the microkeratome

This machine is responsible for creating the perfect (or imperfect) corneal flap. Therefore, it is critical that the microkeratome be evaluated thoroughly before it is used. Among other checks, the surgeon must asses the quality of the blade itself and the function of the depth control. Like the cockpit staff before takeoff, the surgeon has a specific checklist which must be run. Every pilot knows that it is better to identify problems while still on firm ground.

THE PROCEDURE

As with PRK, you are welcomed into the laser suite, and made comfortable on the dentist-type chair. The eye which will undergo the procedure is identified, while your other eye is protected with a shield. Drops are instilled in your eye, including a topical anaesthetic, antibiotic, and possibly a steroid or NSAID. Pre-operative sedation may be used more liberally in

LASIK as this procedure is less dependent on your eye fixation than PRK.

The lid speculum is then inserted into your eye and proper alignment and centration are established. In order to ensure that the corneal flap is repositioned in exactly the right position post-operatively, alignment markings are made. Using dye, a pattern is drawn on the cornea.

A suction ring is placed on the cornea. When the surgeon is confident that it is well centre, suction is activated. The ring is now adherent to the cornea and fixed in position. Your vision becomes blurry as the vacuum is applied. At this time, the IOP is measured. This is a critical step, since an insufficient elevation of IOP may result in a poor flap. When your surgeon is satisfied, the microkeratome is inserted into the suction ring. The microkeratome is moved forward and backward creating a flap. The suction may then be stopped.

The flap is reflected back, exposing the corneal bed. The laser treatment is performed at this time. Following this, the corneal flap is repositioned with care being given to proper alignment and conformity. When the surgeon is satisfied with adhesion of the flap, the operation is over.

The entire procedure, from sitting down to sitting up, is usually less than fifteen minutes.

POST-OP

The first minute

Vision is often blurry. Conversely there are some patients who cry tears of joy within moments of sitting up. Antibiotic, steroid, and/or lubricating drops are instilled. Depending on your surgeon's preference, your eye may be left open, patched, taped shut, or covered with a transparent shield. You may be asked to lie down with your eyes closed for a short while.

The first hour

The first hour is usually spent in a dream-like montage of concern and relief, optimism and fear, waiting for the severe pain which does not come. Irritation, burning, and tearing are to be expected. Many surgeons elect to see their patients thirty minutes or so after the procedure. Typically, they like to examine the operated eye at the slit lamp. The main reason for this is to ensure that the flap is in satisfactory position. If not, it is usually a simple matter to make the necessary adjustments. When your surgeon is satisfied, you are sent on your way with instructions. As a purely precautionary measure, some surgeons cover the eye with a shield overnight to avoid accidental rubbing and to encourage flap adhesion. Vision is variable, but many patients are thrilled with their vision in the immediate post-operative period.

The first day

The day of the surgery is usually uneventful. The eye should be comfortable, and pain medication may be taken if pain arises.

If the eye is open, you may be impressed with the clarity of vision. Or you may not be. Vision is notoriously variable during the first post-operative day. Most people, high myopes in particular, have much better uncorrected vision than they had pre-operatively. Vision generally improves considerably during the first 24 hours.

It is essential to wear the protective shield and to avoid rubbing or squeezing the eye. Although the flap is well-positioned, the healing process has barely begun at this time. The slightest trauma to the eye may move or disrupt the flap. Drops should be used as prescribed. Usually, this consists of a topical antibiotic, a lubricating drop, and possibly a steroid or NSAID. Most people do not experience significant pain because the epithelium is usually intact (except for the flap circumference which heals within 24 hours). If there is severe pain, the possibility of flap displacement should be entertained.

The first post-operative visit is usually the first or second day after surgery. If your eye had been taped overnight, your doctor removes the patch at this time. It is a good opportunity for your surgeon to make sure that everything is healing appropriately. In particular, the flap is examined carefully, as the majority of flap displacements happen in the first day or two following surgery.

Visual acuity, when measured at the first visit, is usually in the 20/30 to 20/60 range. This is somewhat variable and depends a great deal on the pre-operative refractive error. Best corrected vision is often reduced at this visit.

This, however, tends to resolve over time.

The first month

Unlike the post-operative course of PRK, the follow-up appointments are less frequent. There is no need to be seen on a daily basis early on, as the epithelium is intact from 24 hours after surgery. You may be checked about one week after surgery. Then, if everything is going well, you will be seen around the one month mark.

The antibiotic eye drops are discontinued after the first week, as are the steroids if they were used. In fact, if everything is going well, there may be no need to use any eye drops after the first post-operative week.

The eye should be comfortable, and any irritation which was present soon after surgery should have resolved.

By the time the first month has elapsed, vision should be good. Uncorrected as well as best-corrected visual acuity should be reaching the expected levels. The refraction is becoming relatively stable and the success of the initial surgery may be accurately assessed at this time. If it is apparent that the eye is undercorrected, it is appropriate to consider and plan retreatment. Documented stability must be achieved before actually doing enhancement surgery.

The first year

By the three month mark, the office-measured visual acuity has stabilized in most patients. From a qualitative standpoint, some people report continued improvement of their vision beyond that time frame. Subjective problems such as glare and night vision may gradually resolve over periods up to six months.

RESULTS

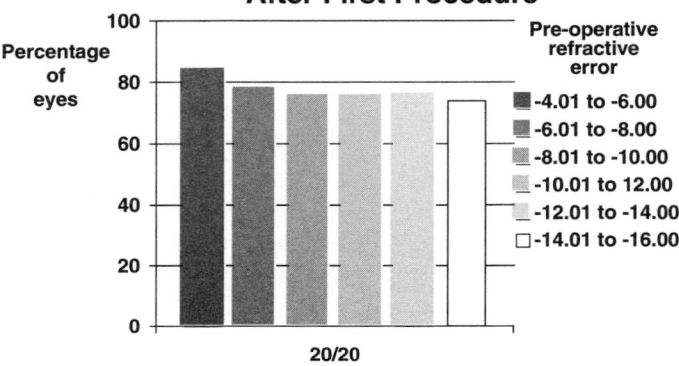

LASIK
Surgical Results for Myopia <u>without</u> Astigmatism
After First Procedure

Pre-operative refractive error
- -4.01 to -6.00
- -6.01 to -8.00
- -8.01 to -10.00
- -10.01 to 12.00
- -12.01 to -14.00
- -14.01 to -16.00

20/20

Post-operative uncorrected visual acuity

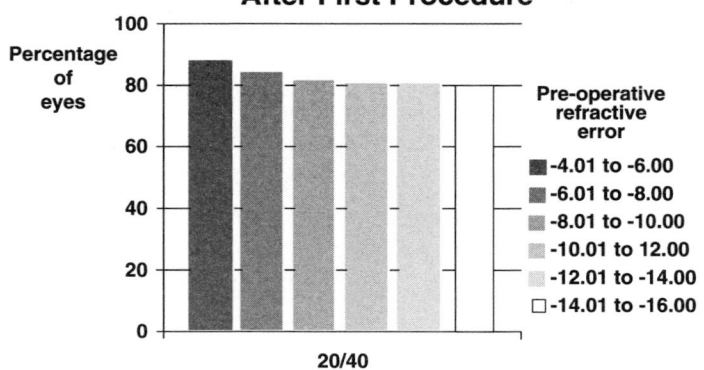

LASIK
Surgical Results for Myopia <u>without</u> Astigmatism
After First Procedure

Pre-operative refractive error
- -4.01 to -6.00
- -6.01 to -8.00
- -8.01 to -10.00
- -10.01 to 12.00
- -12.01 to -14.00
- -14.01 to -16.00

20/40

Post-operative uncorrected visual acuity

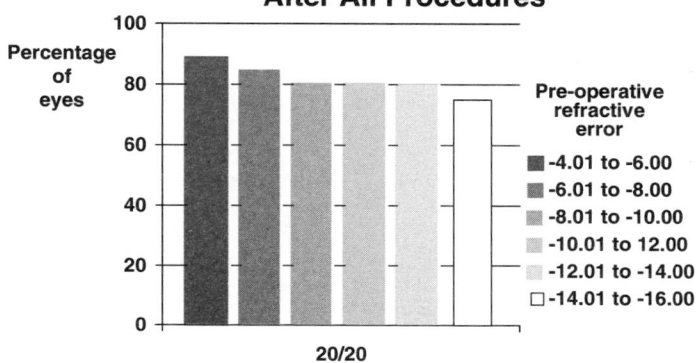

LASIK
Surgical Results for Myopia <u>without</u> Astigmatism
After All Procedures

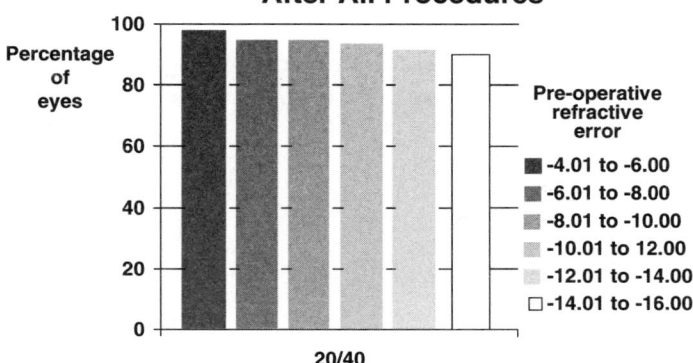

LASIK
Surgical Results for Myopia <u>without</u> Astigmatism
After All Procedures

LASIK
Surgical Results for Myopia <u>without</u> Astigmatism
Within ± 1.00 D of Intended Correction
After All Procedures

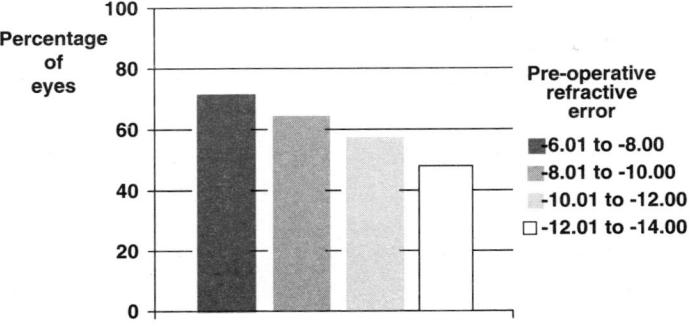

LASIK
Surgical Results for Myopia
Number of Treatments per Eye

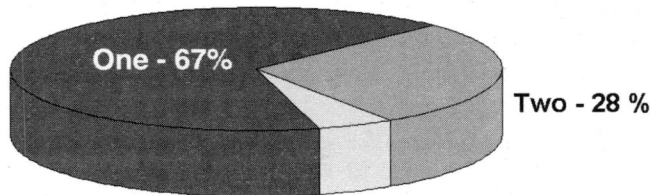

COMPLICATIONS

Undercorrections

As with any form of refractive surgery, undercorrections are seen with LASIK.

Why? The same factors, both known and unknown, that chip away at a 100% predictability, are at work in LASIK.

Numbers: Conservative treatment algorithms, in conjunction with the use of LASIK for higher refractive errors, result in an initial undercorrection rate of 10% to 20%.

Treatment: As always, conservative measure should be attempted first. If they prove unsuccessful, surgical intervention may be advisable.

If? As with PRK, retreatment should not be taken lightly. A second surgical procedure is a whole new ballgame and the risks must be factored into the equation. Just because the first procedure went flawlessly does not ensure that the same thing will happen again. The risks, however, are usually decreased, but may be increased, depending on the specific procedure. Your qualitative vision should be sufficiently poor that the potential benefits outweigh the potential risks. A reasonable cutoff is at the 20/40 range, but the actual standard should be individualized between the patient and the surgeon. Once again, goals of treatment should be specifically defined.

When? Retreatment can be scheduled at any time. The choice of procedure and chances of success are somewhat dependent on timing. Early in the post-operative period, it is possible to lift the flap and repeat the laser treatment in the original stromal bed. This is usually possible until the 12 month mark. Retreatment with LASIK may be considered after this time. At this point, it will most likely be necessary to fashion a brand new flap. In general, it is premature to perform retreatment prior to three months, as the refraction is somewhat labile for this period of time.

How? If a second surgery is required, there are alternatives. Either LASIK may be repeated, or another procedure may be performed.

LASIK after LASIK: Usually this is the best idea. If LASIK was considered to be the best procedure in the first place, chances are it remains the surgery of choice. Unless there were complications with the initial procedure, LASIK enhancement has several advantages. The patient and surgeon are familiar with the outcome of the procedure and the complications of the alternatives are not encountered. And most importantly, the original flap can often be used, which eliminates all of the complications associated with the microkeratome cut. In other words, many of the risks of the first surgery are not a factor in the retreatment. If, however, the original flap is too adherent, another flap may need to be created. The procedure and associated risks are then the same as the original, where a microkeratome is used to fashion a new flap.

PRK after LASIK: This is a valid alternative, however laser ablation of the epithelium must be employed, because there is a risk of flap disruption if the epithelium is removed mechanically. Again, sufficient time should elapse before this procedure is undertaken.

RK after LASIK: It is possible to perform RK after LASIK, but there must be sufficient healing time allowed before the attempt. Performing RK cuts with a poorly adherent flap would increase the risks.

Prognosis: The visual prognosis of undercorrected eyes is excellent.

Overcorrection

Post-operative hyperopia may be seen after myopic LASIK.

Why? The inherent unpredictability of any refractive surgery is again the culprit.

<u>Numbers:</u> Because of the constantly improving conservative treatment algorithms, significant overcorrection is uncommon and decreasing in frequency.

<u>Treatment:</u> Aiming low to avoid overcorrection is the key. Just like bidding for that showcase showdown, the closest to the target without going over is often the winner.

As with PRK, the treatment depends on the extent of overcorrection as well as the age of the patient. If conservative measures are unsuccessful, surgical retreatment is usually of benefit. The procedures themselves are reviewed in the section on hyperopia (See Chapter 10).

<u>Prognosis:</u> The visual prognosis for overcorrected eyes is very good.

Intraoperative flap problems

The most technically challenging component of LASIK is the creation of the flap. As with any learning process, whether it is juggling, snowboarding, or operating, most problems happen early in the learning curve. As the surgeon gains experience, the rate of these flap-related complications drops dramatically to less than 1%. The most serious of these is corneal perforation. This should not occur anywhere along the learning curve, with newer instrument design and proper assembly. Specific problems which may be encountered are summarized.

Small flap: The microkeratome does not advance far enough, causing an incomplete flap to be formed.

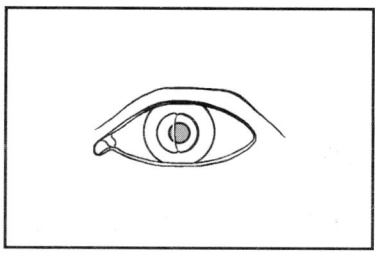

<u>Why?</u> There are a multitude of reasons why this occurs, including microkeratome malfunction, surgeon misjudgment, breakdown of surgical technique, and different eye/orbit variations. The microkeratome is a precision instrument, with narrow limits of tolerance, which demands that all surgical components function accurately and flawlessly.

<u>Treatment:</u> Performing the laser treatment when the cut is too short is risky. Most often, the best answer is to reposition the flap without using the laser. Once the eye has healed in a few months, the procedure may be reattempted. Another option is to enlarge the corneal flap, however this must be done manually at this stage. The lack of precision, when comparing a surgeon's hand to a microkeratome, is a factor which makes this alternative inadvisable unless the cut is past the pupillary edge and almost complete.

<u>Prognosis:</u> There is an excellent visual prognosis if conservative management is employed. When it comes time for the second attempt, it is important to be aware of the reason why the small flap occurred the first time. If the problem was related to the eye and orbital anatomy, it may be worth considering other forms of treatment, such as PRK, to minimize the chance of recurrence.

Free cap: When used in the context of time, speech, and lunch, the word free implies a good thing. Less so in ALK and LASIK. The problem here is that the cut is too long (in relation to the diameter of the flap). The microkeratome does not stop in time to leave a hinge. Therefore, instead of a hinged flap, an unattached cap is created.

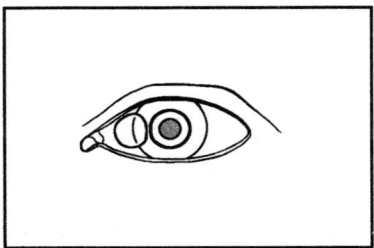

<u>Why?</u> This complication may result for a number of reasons, including microkeratome assembly error. There is an increased incidence of free cap formation in certain eyes, notably those with relatively flat-shaped corneas. Recognition of this risk factor is important in prevention.

<u>Treatment:</u> Once a cap has been formed, there is no point in stopping the procedure. That's like turning around three quarters of the way into an English Channel swim. Proceeding full speed ahead, the laser should be performed as scheduled. Meanwhile, the free cap is stored in a special chamber which has a controlled environment to prevent drying. When the laser treatment has been completed, the cap is repositioned on the stromal bed. It is in this delicate situation where the importance of the alignment markers is truly appreciated.

<u>Prognosis:</u> A little more care and concern may be in order, but unless the cap is damaged, an excellent result can be expected.

Perforated flap: If the microkeratome cut is too superficial, the flap may be thin

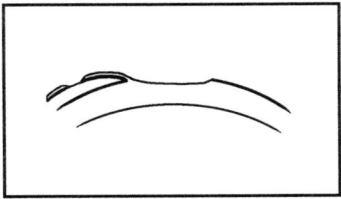

or even perforated.

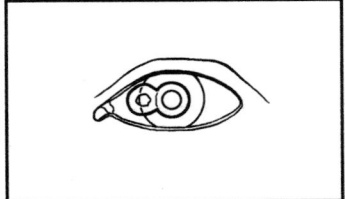

<u>Why?</u> The problem may be related to microkeratome error, or the suction ring losing its attachment to the eye. Of particular importance is the confirmation of adequate IOP before the cut is made. In some eyes, particularly those which have had previous surgery, it is more difficult to obtain and maintain adequate suction, and therefore, adequate intraocular pressure.

<u>Treatment:</u> Recognition of the perforation is the first step. Once this problem has been identified, the procedure should be aborted. The flap should be repositioned and allowed to heal. Subsequent approaches should take into account the reasons for the perforation, and alternative surgery, possibly PRK, should be considered. Retreatment should be delayed for several months to allow healing to occur. In extenuating circumstances, if the perforation is small, the surgeon may elect to proceed cautiously with the procedure.

<u>Prognosis:</u> The results are variable, depending on the degree and location of the perforation. A small, eccentric flap hole may allow excellent surgical results, either initially or upon retreatment. Other more complicated cases may result in the loss of best-corrected visual acuity.

Corneal perforation: As opposed to a flap perforation, this refers to a corneal incision which is too deep and violates the stromal bed, creating a communication between the inside of the eye and the outside world.

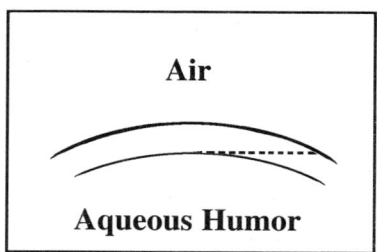

<u>Why?</u> This is a serious problem which only happens when there has been a serious error. The depth controlling device is either set incorrectly or has not been inserted. This allows the

microkeratome to cut deeper than it should. It is also possible that the cornea itself was too thin, but that problem is specifically screened for using pre-operative pachymetry.

<u>Treatment:</u> In this instance, prevention can not be overstated. Pre-operative checks, when done appropriately and meticulously, make this potentially catastrophic event impossible. If corneal perforation does occur, management may require all of the surgeon's expertise and experience.

<u>Prognosis:</u> A hole in the eye is not a good thing at the best of times, and when the IOP has been increased by the suction ring, this is certainly not the best of times. At the risk of being too graphic, imagine a water balloon filled with water. If you increase the pressure by squeezing it then suddenly puncture the balloon with a knife, you may find yourself in need of a towel. The corresponding ocular condition is the expulsion of intraocular contents. This is a severe, sight-threatening problem which cannot occur with proper assembly of the instrument. It has been reported only rarely.

Subconjunctival hemorrhage

The eye is red post-operatively.

<u>Why?</u> The suction ring, on occasion, may disrupt tiny subconjunctival blood vessels. The white of the eye may have one or two deep red spots and people may ask you what the other person looked like.

<u>Treatment:</u> There is no specific treatment.

<u>Prognosis:</u> There is no pain or significant consequences of a subconjunctival hemorrhage. Things gradually return to normal over the following couple of weeks.

Pain

The majority of patients do not complain of post-operative pain. There is often some irritation, burning, or mild discomfort.

Why? Any time an eye undergoes an operation, it is quite natural that it is more sensitive. Pain after LASIK is quite unusual because the epithelium remains intact. When severe pain does occur, it may be in the context of flap displacement or epithelial defect.

Numbers: Significant pain is seen infrequently, about 2% in LASIK, compared with 10% in PRK. The time course is similar. The first day is the worst.

Treatment: Mild discomfort during the initial post-operative period may be treated with painkillers, however most patients find lubricating drops adequate. In the event of an epithelial defect or flap displacement, these problems should be addressed directly.

Displaced flap

Occasionally, the corneal flap may become dislodged in the first few hours post-operatively.

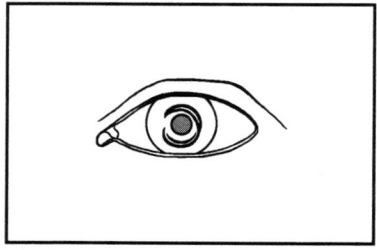

Why? The forces holding the flap in position are relatively weak in the immediate post-operative period. It takes 12 to 24 hours for the flap edges to heal over, and months for the cornea to regain most of its pre-operative structural integrity. During the first day, even minor forces such as eyelid squeezing may displace the flap. As time goes by and the cornea heals, the eye is less threatened by minor, and even major, trauma.

Numbers: The chances of this complication are greatest in the first twenty-four hours, however delayed displacement may occur in conjunction with eye trauma. Overall, the chance of suffering a displaced flap is less than 1%.

Treatment: It is not difficult to make the diagnosis. The eye is irritated and may be red, the patient may be in pain, and the vision is blurred, having not improved over the first few hours as expected. The flap is displaced and the surgeon is the rocket scientist who pieces it all together. Management of this complication involves repositioning the flap quickly and accurately.

Prognosis: Unless the flap has been displaced too long and has developed wrinkles, visual prognosis is good.

Epithelial defects

Many of the advantages which LASIK offers over PRK are conferred because no epithelial defect is created in the former. Usually.

Why? Mechanical trauma, drug sensitivity, and predisposition of the eye all play a role.

Numbers: In a small number of patients (1% to 2%), there is an epithelial defect. Most frequently this is seen in the immediate post-operative period.

Treatment: The treatment of this condition is similar to the post-operative management of PRK eyes. Medications, including antibiotics and anti-inflammatory eye drops, are prescribed. In addition, a bandage contact lens may promote healing and reduce pain. Patients should be seen frequently to assess healing and watch for infection and flap displacement.

Prognosis: Epithelial defects usually heal in a quick and uncomplicated fashion. Infections develop rarely. Of concern in LASIK are the potential long-term consequences of this complication. It appears that the risk of epithelial ingrowth (described later) may be increased in eyes with a post-operative epithelial defect.

Corneal Infection

Any time an eye meets a surgeon, there is a theoretical risk of infection.

> Why? The difference in infection rates is attributable to the post-operative epithelial defect which is created in PRK and not usually seen in LASIK. When the epithelium is not intact, the cornea is more susceptible to bacterial invasion.

> Numbers: With modern day technology and techniques, surgical infections in elective procedures are rare. The chance of an infection is low in PRK, around one in a thousand. In LASIK, the odds are even better, on the order of one in five thousand.

> Treatment: An eye with a corneal infection is often red, painful, and demonstrates a reduction in visual acuity. Examination reveals an area of whitening on the cornea. There is often evidence of sympathetic inflammation within the eye itself. Treatment, as in a post-PRK infection, consists of aggressive antibiotic therapy.

> Prognosis: Depending on the severity, a corneal infection may have devastating effects. Vision often drops suddenly and the amount of recovery is variable. In the best case scenario, the infection is mild, peripheral, and responds well to treatment. The result may be just a mild, visually insignificant corneal scar and 20/20 vision. Other patients may not be so fortunate and significant visual loss may occur.

Night glare

The halos and difficulty with night vision are seen with LASIK, just as in PRK.

> Why? The culprit, once again, is often the limited treatment zone. If the pupil dilates larger than the optical zone, night glare may arise. Early in the healing process, some halo effect may occur.

Numbers: In mild to moderate myopes, these symptoms are less of a problem, because larger treatment zones are possible. As higher levels of myopia are treated, the treatment zone diameter becomes limited. Consequently, such visual disturbances become increasingly common.

Treatment/Prognosis: The majority of these problems will resolve as the healing process takes place. As time goes by, patients become more accustomed to their vision. An enhancement procedure may be attempted if the problem is persistent and severe.

Epithelial ingrowth

Epithelial cell which normally reside on the front of the cornea, may decide to grow under the flap.

Why? In PRK, epithelial cells have nowhere to go but back to their usual home on the surface of the cornea. In LASIK, a cut has been made in the cornea. These cells can now migrate between the flap and the stromal bed and set up shop at the interface.

Numbers: On average, this occurs in 1% to 2% of eyes following LASIK. Most often this is seen in the first few weeks after the procedure. Eyes with a post-operative epithelial defect are predisposed to develop this complication, as are eyes with a perforated flap.

Treatment: Diagnosis is made when whitish epithelium is observed at the flap interface. Management depends on the severity of symptoms, the size and location of the ingrowth, and whether it is progressive or static. Treatment, when necessary, involves lifting the flap and removing the transplanted epithelium.

Prognosis: The ultimate effect of this complication is variable, depending on factors such as location and size. If managed early, good vision may be preserved, but if not, an epithelial ingrowth may cause damage to the overlying flap resulting in a *stromal melt*. When this happens, the situation becomes more complicated and the visual prognosis is worse. Therefore, early recognition and treatment are vital.

Myopic Regression

Regression toward myopia may be seen after LASIK.

Why? When the cornea heals, the effect of the surgery may be partially diminished.

Numbers: When the corneal stroma is excised or lasered at a depth, it is less reactive than the superficial layers. Myopic regression, therefore, is usually a little less severe following LASIK than after PRK. To some degree, this phenomenon is seen in 100% of cases. However, in high myopes, the severity of the regression increases. Stabilization usually occurs earlier in LASIK, as the surface healing process is fast-forwarded. Typically, most regression is noted in the first three months.

Treatment/Prognosis: Topical steroids are less effective in regression following LASIK than in post-PRK regression. If visually significant regression occurs, retreatment may be necessary. Alternatively, consideration may be given to monovision.

Retinal hemorrhages

Hemorrhages in the retina have been observed post-operatively.

Why? The most likely explanation is the elevation in IOP which is induced intraoperatively.

Numbers: This phenomenon is observed uncommonly.

Treatment: There is no specific treatment for retinal hemorrhages. Most often, they disappear by themselves over time.

Prognosis: Unless the hemorrhages are obscuring the central macula, the vision is not usually affected. Theoretically, a severe or unfortunately located hemorrhage could have visual significance.

Others

Ptosis, irregular astigmatism, dryness, irritation, and decentration may also be seen following LASIK.

LASIK Summary

Advantages:

- Quick visual rehabilitation
- Minimal pain
- Epithelium remains intact
- Superior results for high myopia
- Long-term eye drops not required
- Less myopic regression than RK, PRK
- May be used effectively in myopia *and* hyperopia

Disadvantages:

- Precision instrumentation required (in addition to the laser)
- Technically difficult to perform
- Risk of flap-related problems
- Long-term studies not available
- FDA approval pending (LASIK)

Best in...

High Myopes: People with myopia greater than -9 D have always had a higher incidence of haze and regression following PRK. In this subset of people, RK and PRK have demonstrated less acceptable complication rates. LASIK was specifically designed for these individuals and the results are encouraging.

<u>The Need for Speed</u>: One of the biggest advantages of LASIK is the quick visual recovery. It is ideal for people with occupational reasons to minimize down time.

<u>Simultaneous Bilateral Surgery</u> : There are two reasons why this subset of people may do better with LASIK. The first is that their vision immediately post-operatively should be better than with PRK. This is nice in unilateral cases, but a huge advantage when both eyes are done simultaneously. Instead of lying around the house for the first few days, patients may have useful vision from day one. The second reason is that a bilateral LASIK may be less risky than a bilateral RK or PRK. The reason is that most of the big risks with LASIK occur *during* the procedure. Therefore, if one eye is operated on and everything goes fine, the patient and surgeon can feel comfortable moving on to the second eye. In contrast, the major risks of PRK occur post-operatively, so you're not out of the woods the moment that the first eye is done.

<u>Gain Without Pain</u>: Because of the reduced incidence and severity of post-operative pain, LASIK is well suited for those who are reluctant to leave their pain-free environment.

<u>After RK</u>: In specific situations, LASIK may be preferable to PRK for people who have had RK which has left them myopic or hyperopic.

<u>Impaired Wound Healing</u>: Patients with the potential for abnormal wound healing may do better with LASIK because re-epithelialization of the cornea is not required.

<u>Eye drop intolerance</u>: Nobody likes taking eye drops. There are patients, however, who are bothered sufficiently that they are unable to bring an eye drop container within five feet of their eye. Also, there are individuals who have previously taken eye drops and are known to react adversely. This is most significant in "steroid responders" whose IOP's rise after long-term use of topical steroids. Because eye drops are generally used for only a short period of time after LASIK, this procedure may be advisable for such drug intolerant surgical candidates.

High astigmatism: LASIK may be a better, safer procedure for individuals with high degrees of astigmatism

Mild and moderate myopes? In some hands, the results of LASIK are very good. So good, that some surgeons believe that LASIK should be used not only for high myopes, but also for mild and moderate myopes. They see LASIK as a technically superior procedure with less drawbacks and equal or better results. In fact, some proponents of LASIK publicly labelled the much anticipated FDA approval of PRK a 'stillbirth'. They suggested that PRK was out of date even before it arrived. Currently, there is a debate in the ophthalmic community about whether LASIK should replace PRK as the treatment of choice in mild and moderate myopes.

7

RADIAL
KERATOTOMY (RK)

THE ROAD TO 1997

It was almost one hundred years ago that a surgeon from the Netherlands performed his first refractive surgery experiments on rabbits. He came to the conclusion that making incisions in their corneas served to flatten them.

In 1933, a Japanese surgeon learned a lesson from Mother Nature. One of his patients who had a disease known as keratoconus, developed a tear in Descemet's layer of the cornea. This doctor observed that once the eye had healed, the cornea was flatter and the vision was improved. This led him to embark on a series of experiments using corneal incisions to alter the refraction.

The baton was passed to a Russian surgeon who also attended the Mother Nature School of Ophthalmology. A myopic man suffered a lacerated cornea when his glasses shattered in a fight. After the eye healed, this patient was found to have better uncorrected vision than before. The doctor concluded that the shape of the cornea was flatter after the accident, which inadvertently

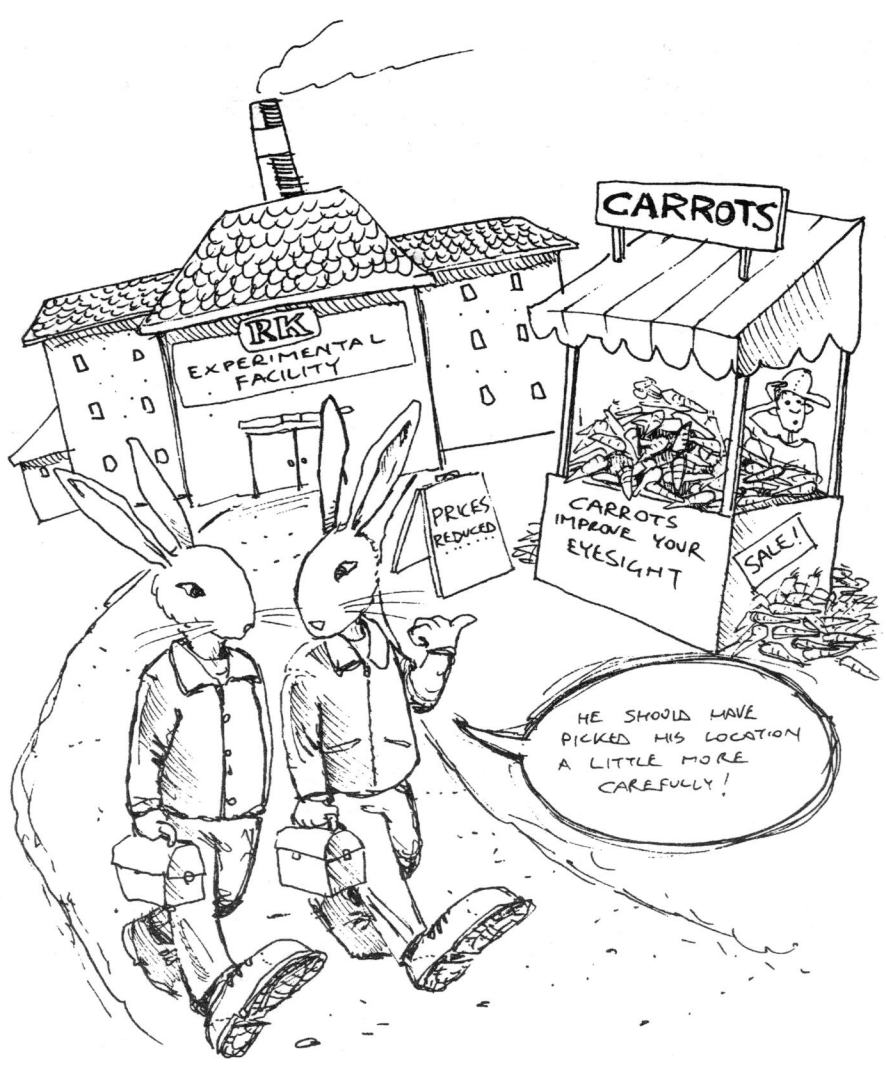

cured the myopia.

The art of RK was brought from Moscow to the United States in 1978. Early procedures sparked media and public interest, and also a controversy about the safety and efficacy of RK. Large scale studies have been performed in the hope of addressing these questions. Since its infancy, RK has been performed in over two million patients worldwide, and the procedure itself has evolved a great deal.

IS RK FOR YOU?

RK may be used to correct a wide range of myopia. The results, however, are dependent on the degree of pre-operative myopia. At the current time, RK is generally reserved for the treatment of mild to moderate myopia. Contraindications are similar to those for PRK and LASIK.

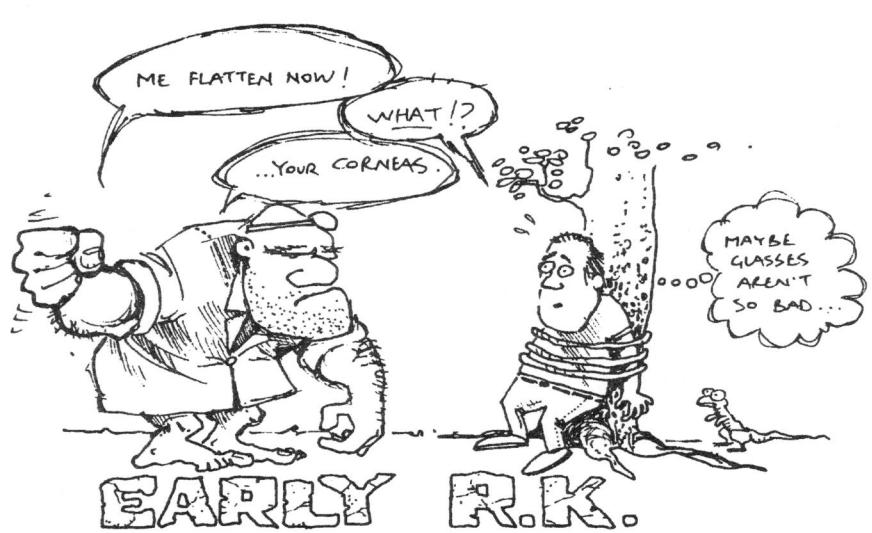

THE PROCEDURE

The pre-operative evaluation and preparation are similar for RK as for PRK and LASIK.

The procedure is performed under topical anaesthesia and you may be offered pre-operative sedation. After centring the eye, partial thickness radial cuts are made in the cornea with a diamond knife. This allows the corneal curvature to relax, resulting in a flatter refractive surface. The central part of the cornea, the visual axis, is left untouched. The procedure takes about twenty minutes.

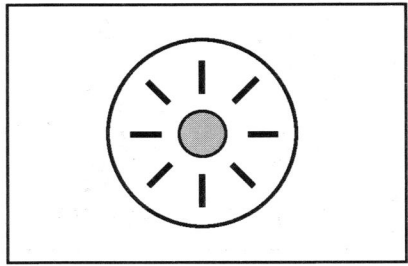

From experiments and experience, ophthalmologists know that certain variables must be taken into account when performing RK.

Number of incisions. More cuts cause more effect. Higher myopes require a greater number of incisions. The effect is not proportional, however. Eight cuts do not give twice as much refractive change as four incisions. In fact, the majority of the work is done by the first four cuts. The idea is to perform the minimum amount of surgery that will accomplish the goal and the range is usually between four and sixteen cuts.

Depth of incisions. Deeper cuts cause more effect. In order to achieve adequate results, the incision depths are usually on the order of 90% corneal thickness.

Optical zone. The greater the myopia, the closer the incisions must be to the visual axis. In someone with severe myopia, the untreated central optical zone will be smaller than in a mild myope. Typical incisions are 3 to 4 mm in length.

Age. As people get older, RK has greater effect. A forty year old eye will require less aggressive treatment than an identical eye in a twenty year old.

Sex. The eyes of females do not tend to respond as much to RK as those of males. This effect is exaggerated in younger people. Therefore, a twenty-year old female's eye will require more aggressive treatment than an identical eye in her twin brother.

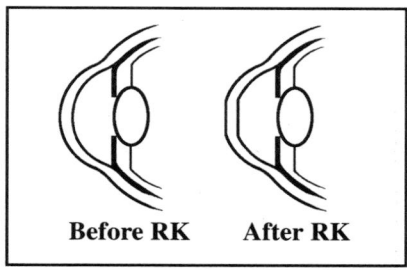

Before RK   After RK

POST-OP

The first day

Once the anaesthetic wears off, you feel like there is something in your eye. Usually there is no significant pain, just this sensation. Uncorrected vision in the immediate post-operative period is customarily good, and most often far better than your vision would have been at one day post-PRK. Antibiotic eye drops are prescribed. The surgeon usually checks the eye on the day after surgery for a routine examination.

The first week

The foreign body sensation disappears within a few days. The vision gradually improves, although it may fluctuate considerably throughout the day. The antibiotic eye drops are used for about a week after surgery, at which time your ophthalmologist may check you once again. You may be reminded to wear protective eyewear when engaging in potentially dangerous activities.

The first month

The eye is comfortable and the vision is good. Fluctuating vision and/or glare symptoms may be the only things reminding you that you had surgery. A post-operative visit to your doctor around the one month mark is not unusual.

The first year

Fluctuating vision and glare symptoms usually improve as time goes by. You may notice your crystal clear vision deteriorating somewhat if you are the victim of a hyperopic shift (described later). You continue to wear protective eyewear as a precautionary measure, when the situation warrants it.

RESULTS

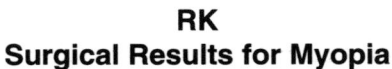

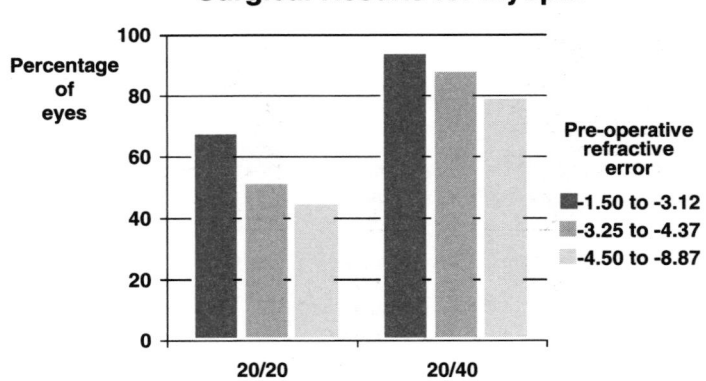

RK
Surgical Results for Myopia

Percentage of eyes

Pre-operative refractive error
■ -1.50 to -3.12
▨ -3.25 to -4.37
▢ -4.50 to -8.87

Post-operative uncorrected visual acuity

RK
Surgical Results for Myopia
Number of Treatments per Eye

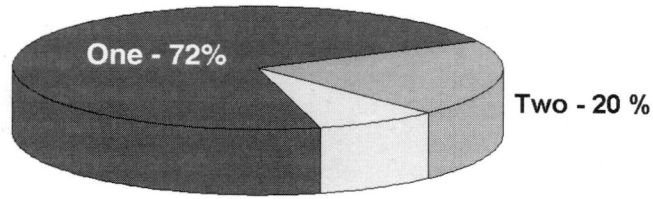

One - 72%

Two - 20 %

Three or more - 8 %

RK
Selected Complications

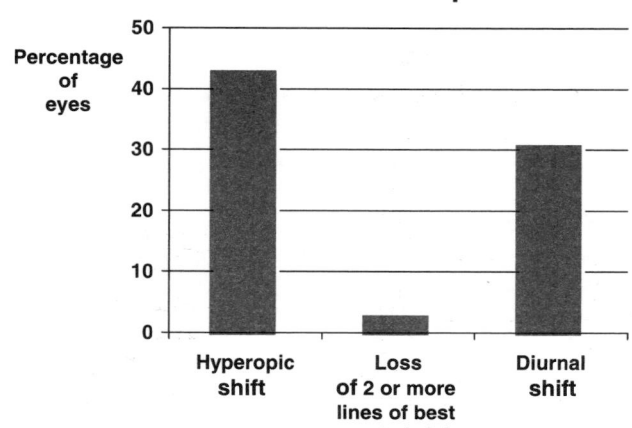

Percentage of eyes

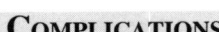

COMPLICATIONS

Undercorrections

Post-operative residual myopia may be seen following RK.

Why? The inherent imprecision of any refractive procedure comes into play.

Numbers: Long term RK data suggests that 25% of RK patients will remain myopic.

Treatment: Conservative treatment is usually warranted in the initial post-operative period. Still, a significant percentage of people who undergo RK are left with a residual refractive error and consider retreatment.

If? As with PRK and LASIK, a second surgery should not be undertaken casually. Risks, benefits, and goals should be clearly addressed pre-operatively.

When? Stability of the eye should be documented before proceeding with retreatment.

How? Until recently, the options for undercorrected patients were to have RK enhancement, or to grin and bear it. With the development of the excimer laser, many former RK patients are looking to this new technology for a solution. Once a cornea has been operated on, whether under the knife or the laser, it is important to recognize that it is now different. This class of eyes, therefore, must be evaluated as a separate group.

RK after RK: If enhancement is necessary, RK may be used to supplement the original procedure. More corneal incisions may be made, usually to a maximum of 16. The effect of this second round of radial cuts is predictably less than the effect of the first attempt. Alternatively, the original incisions may be deepened or lengthened.

PRK after RK: There is no clear answer regarding the

effectiveness and safety of PRK after RK. The numbers are relatively small, but certain trends are emerging. The overall results are more variable than after the original surgery. Some studies suggest that the success levels are comparable to PRK on virgin eyes, but other research reveals a higher rate of post-operative refractive errors. Although some patients are thrilled with perfect results, others may not be so fortunate. In addition, there may be an increased potential for complications in these eyes. Specifically, there may be a greater possibility of post-operative corneal haze, which could cause a reduction in best-corrected visual acuity. While further treatments may be necessary, it appears that, despite the increased risks, good results may be obtained. This is especially true with new laser delivery systems and techniques.

LASIK after RK: There is even less information about this approach, but the news is encouraging. The post-operative epithelial haze seen with PRK is virtually nonexistent. In addition, the predictability of LASIK following RK, seems to be superior to PRK. However, LASIK is not without its risks. After RK, the corneal flap may behave differently. In fact, in rare cases, the resulting flap edge consists of a number of pie-shaped segments, which correspond to the RK incisions. This is not good, not common, but not to be forgotten. In spite of this small risk, it appears that LASIK may be a better procedure than PRK in the treatment of undercorrected RK.

Prognosis: The final visual results, after initial undercorrection, are excellent.

Overcorrection

Hyperopia following RK may be seen.

Why? The numerous variables which we know, combined with the infinite variables which we do not control, contribute to the unpredictability of RK. In addition, the hyperopic shift (described later) contributes to progressive hyperopia in those who are not overcorrected initially.

<u>Numbers:</u> Long term RK data suggests that one third of RK patients will end up hyperopic.

<u>Treatment:</u> Once again, just as with haircuts and toast, it is better to be underdone than overdone. Prevention of overcorrection is paramount. As with the other forms of refractive surgery, the decision to treat the hyperopia should be based upon the risks and benefits of conservative and aggressive management. The techniques for the treatment of hyperopia are addressed in Chapter 10.

<u>Prognosis:</u> Effective retreatment methods provide a very good visual prognosis.

Hyperopic shift

Long-term studies have revealed a phenomenon known as the hyperopic shift. An eye which was perfectly corrected to plano six months after surgery, may continue a slow drift toward hyperopia. This is in contrast to myopic regression which takes the eye back to where it started.

<u>Why?</u> Corneal instability is thought to be the culprit. RK incisions cause flattening of the cornea to continue for years after the surgery.

<u>Numbers:</u> Anywhere from 20 to 50% of eyes may demonstrate this shift. This is most pronounced in the first few years after RK, where 0.5 D of hyperopia may affect a previously plano eye. The hyperopic shift has been documented up to ten years after the surgery. On average, about 5% of eyes encounter a significant hyperopic shift every year after RK.

<u>Treatment:</u> If the hyperopia is tolerated well, there is no reason for aggressive treatment. Eyestrain symptoms may result, especially in older, presbyopic individuals. Glasses are an option, as are surgical techniques. Various procedures have been

suggested, including PRK, ALK, and LASIK, and these procedures will be reviewed in Chapter 10.

Hyperopic shift was the reason behind the development of a modified RK technique. Minimally invasive radial keratotomy or Mini-RK is just what it sounds like. A version of RK which is less aggressive and, in theory, has less side effects. Mini-RK is similar to RK, except that it involves shorter (2 to 3 mm) and fewer (2 to 4) incisions. This is a relatively new technique, but initial indications suggest that it is effective for mild myopia yet does not exhibit the troublesome hyperopic shift.

Prognosis: Surgical treatment of hyperopia is more difficult in an eye which has had RK. Good results are still possible with cautious surgical care.

Perforations/Microperforations

The difference is one of extent, where a microperforation usually refers to a self-sealing full thickness corneal laceration less than 1 mm in length. True perforations are larger wounds which may be associated with loss of aqueous fluid and collapse of the anterior chamber.

Why? When a knife is cutting at 90% depths, there is not much cornea left between the blade and the inside of the eye. All in all, it would not be a good time for an earthquake.

Numbers: Although higher numbers have been reported in the past, technological improvements have dropped the incidence of microperforations to approximately 2% to 4%. True perforations with aqueous fluid leakage and collapse of the anterior chamber are rare.

Treatment: The importance of a microperforation lies in its recognition. If it goes undetected and the incision extended, it may become a true perforation. An uncomplicated microperforation is often merely observed. Suturing is only necessary if there is persistent leakage. Antibiotics and a bandage contact lens may be used, and post-operative checks may be more frequent. True perforations are managed more aggressively and suturing may be necessary to close the wound.

Prognosis: Serious sequelae from microperforations are rare. True perforations are really penetrating intraocular wounds and should be considered sight threatening.

Excursions into the optical zone

An incision can occasionally extend into the clear optical zone.

Why? RK is a manual, technically challenging procedure. For any number of reasons, the knife may extend the incision toward the visual axis.

Numbers: Excursions may be as small as 0.25 mm and as large as the eye. Usually, the incisions encroach only slightly on the clear optical zone. Overall, the incidence is approximately 1%.

Treatment: Just like a broken promise, an extended incision is impossible to undo. Prevention is the key.

Prognosis: Fortunately, persistent symptoms are uncommon. Occasionally, glare symptoms may result from excursions.

Irregular astigmatism

Regular or irregular astigmatism may remain after RK or be induced by RK.

Why? RK alone (without AK-See Chapter 7) will usually not reduce the amount of astigmatism. In addition, healing may occur in an irregular pattern which may result in post-operative astigmatism.

Numbers: Small amounts of astigmatism, that is less than 1 D, are not uncommon post-operatively. This is usually a visually insignificant problem. Uncommonly, larger astigmatic errors may be encountered. This is most often seen in patients with moderate or severe pre-operative refractive errors who required more aggressive surgery.

Treatment: Glasses or contact lenses may be attempted, however further surgery may be considered once the eye has stabilized.

Prognosis: Most often, astigmatism is adequately managed and satisfactory vision results. On occasion, irregular astigmatism may be refractory to treatment and may cause a decrease in best-corrected visual acuity.

Glare, light sensitivity, starbursts

A variety of visual phenomena may be seen following RK, even in eyes with 20/20 vision.

Why? When the pupil enlarges at night, the peripheral corneal incisions come into play. If the RK scars encroach on the pupil, peripheral light rays may cause a variety of unwanted visual symptoms.

Numbers: The majority of patients experience symptoms of this nature in the immediate post-operative period. In all but a few, however, they disappear spontaneously after a few months. The smaller the optical zone, the greater the risk of these symptoms persisting.

Treatment: Maintenance of a sufficiently large optical zone should prevent persistent problems. Usually no treatment is required for transient glare symptoms. Persistent difficulties are somewhat difficult to treat. Topical steroids and tear drops are sometimes helpful.

Prognosis: Patience in the post-operative period is usually rewarded. The vast majority of these symptoms go away after a few months. An unfortunate few are left with incapacitating night time difficulties.

Infection

Infection of the cornea (corneal ulcer) as well as of the eye itself (endophthalmitis) are risks of RK.

> Why? Any time a cut is made in the cornea, the potential for infection exists. If, in addition, there is a perforation of the globe, there is the theoretical risk that bacteria can invade the eye itself.

> Numbers: The chance of developing a corneal ulcer following RK is less than 1/1000. The chance of endophthalmitis is even less.

> Treatment: Topical antibiotics are the mainstay of management for both of these conditions. Surgery may be required in the event of endophthalmitis.

> Prognosis: These are vision threatening complications. The prognosis is dependent on, among other things, the delay in treatment. Despite appropriate management, there may be some loss of visual acuity.

Globe rupture

There is a theoretical risk of globe rupture following RK.

> Why? Deep corneal incisions may predispose the eye to injury. It makes sense that an eye with RK is weaker than an unoperated eye, at least until the incisions heal. Mild trauma which would otherwise cause insignificant injury, may cause a globe rupture in the post-operative RK eye.

> Numbers: It is rare for an eye to encounter trauma following RK, but it has been reported. The results are somewhat mixed. There are reports of severe, vision threatening injuries to RK eyes. Conversely, there have been post-operative eyes which have withstood trauma. Without performing a cruel and inhumane scientific study, it is difficult to determine the actual risk. Many ophthalmologists do believe that an eye is, in fact, predisposed

to serious injury following RK.

Treatment: It is advisable to avoid injury to the eyes at all times, particularly following RK, and especially in the early post-operative period. Protective eyewear should be worn during sports. Should an accident occur, the management depends on the nature and severity of the injury.

Prognosis: The prognosis depends on the nature and severity of the injury.

Contact lens intolerance

Although it is unusual to have difficulty wearing soft contact lenses after RK, rigid lens wearers often have problems.

Why? The problem is caused by a combination of an increase in corneal sensitivity and a change in corneal curvature.

Treatment: There is no specific treatment for contact lens intolerance. Whether it is related to comfort or fit, it is important to realize pre-operatively that this may happen. Regardless, contact lenses cannot be worn for at least three months following RK.

Prognosis: The prognosis is variable, but better for those who wear soft contact lenses instead of rigid ones.

Fluctuating vision

Following RK, some people complain that their vision fluctuates throughout the day.

Why? The cornea swells up at night and this affects the refractive error of the eye. In the morning, it seems as if the effect of the RK has been accentuated, and the vision is often better. By the evening, when the cornea is relatively dry, the effect of the surgery appears not as noticeable.

<u>Numbers:</u> Many patients experience this symptom following RK. It is most common in the early post-operative period.

<u>Treatment:</u> Patience is the answer, however eye drops which modify the corneal fluid content may be helpful.

<u>Prognosis:</u> Although fluctuating vision may persist for months to years, it gradually becomes less noticeable. It may never disappear entirely, but only rarely does it becomes a debilitating problem.

Others

Other complications include cataract, glaucoma, recurrent corneal erosions, decentration, dryness, irritation, and ptosis.

Summary

Advantages

- **Two million patient track record**
- **Long-term studies available**
- **Predictable effect in low myopes**
- **Visual axis spared**
- **Visual improvement quicker than PRK**

Disadvantages

- **Theoretical post-operative corneal weakness predisposes to injury**
- **Less predictable in high myopes**
- **Hyperopic shift**
- **Risk of globe perforation, intraocular infection**
- **Fluctuating vision**
- **Not effective in hyperopia**

Best in...

Low myopes: The accuracy and safety record of RK is difficult to beat in myopes under 3 D. Unpredictability and complications increase in frequency in moderate and severe myopia.

Impatient patients: The time required for visual improvement is less than after PRK, but likely more than after LASIK.

Cost-conscious eyes: The equipment costs alone are far less than any excimer procedure. This translates into a less expensive fee for RK than for PRK or LASIK.

Technophobia: Some people prefer the train to the airplane. It may not be as futuristic, but it gets you where you want to go. RK, too, will get you where you want to go.

8

Cataract Extraction
Refractive Lensectomy

Cataract Extraction

The most common eye operation in the world today is the cataract extraction. You will recall that a cataract is a cloudiness in the crystalline lens. When it becomes opaque, light is prevented from reaching the retina and vision deteriorates. The logical solution, therefore, is to remove the cataract.

There is a problem, however. The crystalline lens is a powerful tissue. That is, it has diopteric power. As you recall from Chapter 2, the crystalline lens is responsible for a significant amount of refraction. If we then remove it, as is done in a cataract extraction, the eye has lost part of its power, and light is focused behind the eye. This is called an *aphakic* eye.

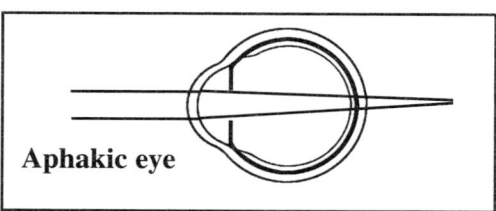

Aphakic eye

In order to focus the light on the retina, this power must be replaced. The best solution is usually an intraocular lens. An eye with an implant is called a *pseudophakic* eye.

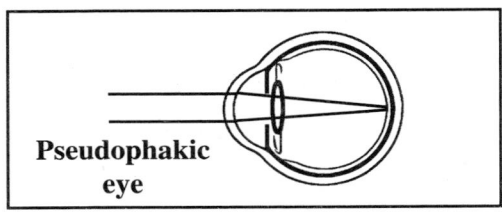

Pseudophakic eye

Among other things, they vary in size, shape, composition, and the exact location within the eye, but the goal is always the same. To implant a lens of the best possible power.

If a cataract is removed from a 5 D myopic eye, and the effective power of the replacement intraocular lens is the same as that of the preoperative crystalline lens, the resulting eye will be 5.00 D myopic. Nothing is different except that the new lens is clearer. However, perhaps this may not be the best possible power for the intraocular lens.

If, however, we implant a lens which has exactly 5.00 D less effective power, then magically the myopia will disappear. Someone who has worn distance glasses for the first eighty years of their life will now be 20/20 uncorrected. Almost makes you wish you had a cataract!

Refractive Lensectomy

People who have hail damaged vehicles get their cars painted. That doesn't mean that you need to drive around in search of a hail storm. If you want your car to be a different color, go ahead and paint it. This same philosophy helped spawn the *refractive lensectomy*. A cataract extraction when there is no cataract. That's all it is. It is exactly the same procedure, only the term *cataract* cannot be used.

There is a bit of a grey area. Many people over the age of forty-five have some

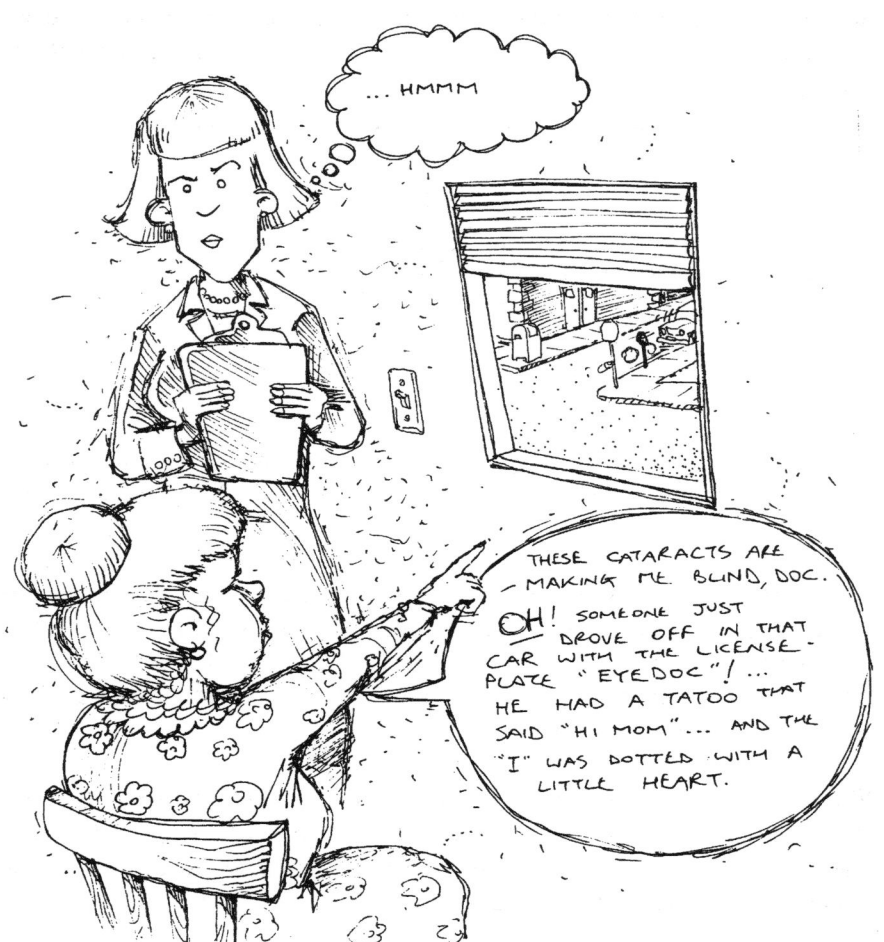

degree of clouding in their crystalline lens. By definition, they have cataracts. However, if the changes are so minor that an individual can see 20/20 despite these "cataracts", then should these really be considered true cataracts? How about a 20/25 "cataract"? Where do you draw the line?

It is basically just a question of semantics. It doesn't really matter what you call it, as long as you understand it. If you're having trouble seeing because of the cataract, then the operation should be called a cataract extraction. If, however, your best-corrected vision is perfect and your cataracts are visually insignificant, then it would be advisable to consider this operation as a refractive lensectomy.

The Procedure

There are three general ways to remove a cataract:

Intracapsular

When your grandparents had their cataracts removed, it was probably by this technique. The whole crystalline lens, including the entire capsule, was removed. It was better than nothing, but this method had its share of problems and risks. Unless there is an exceptional situation, intracapsular cataract extraction would be better off in the history books than in a 1996 operating room.

Extracapsular

Still an acceptable technique today, this procedure makes a hole, or *capsulotomy,* in the anterior capsule. The nucleus of the cataract is expressed through it and the remaining lens material is sucked away with an irrigation/ aspiration device. The posterior capsule is usually preserved, in order to support the posterior chamber intraocular lens (PCIOL).

If the posterior capsule is not preserved, which sometimes happens during an operation, then there are two options. Either a PCIOL can be sutured into place, or an anterior chamber intraocular lens (ACIOL) can be implanted.

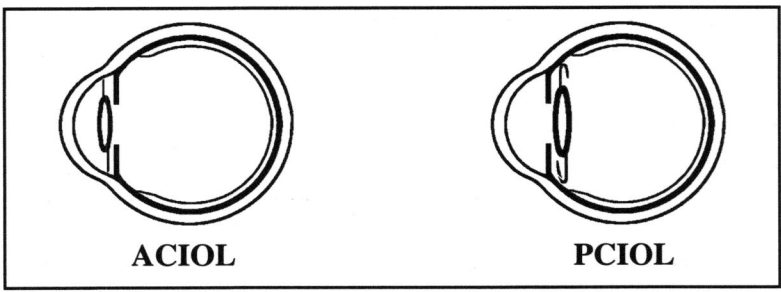

ACIOL   **PCIOL**

Phacoemulsification

This is the newest technique of cataract extraction. A different kind of hole is made in the anterior capsule (a *capsulorhexis*), then a small ultrasound probe is inserted into the eye through a small incision. The vibration of the probe converts a hard cataract into a liquid form which is sucked away by a vacuum. Again, the posterior capsule is generally preserved and a PCIOL is implanted.

There are a few advantages to phacoemulsification. The incision size is smaller. Instead of having to make a 6 mm incision through which to express the nucleus of the cataract, the incision can be half the size. And if the incision is constructed in such a fashion that it is self-sealing, there may be no need to place a suture. The healing time is also less, so post-operative vision improves more quickly. If performed under topical anaesthesia, vision immediately after surgery will be better.

The disadvantage of phacoemulsification is that some surgeons find it more technically challenging than the extracapsular method.

Probably the best advice is to find a surgeon you are comfortable with and have them use technique they perfer.

Anaesthesia

General

Only in unusual situations is it advisable to be "put under" for a cataract extraction. The risks of general anaesthesia, although small, are still significantly greater than the alternatives.

Retrobulbar/Parabulbar

This is the most common form of anaesthesia. A needle injects local anaesthetic around the eye to stop sensation and movement. Usually this is done in conjunction with an intravenous sedative. Although you are awake throughout the procedure, you are sleepy and relaxed. Immediately after the procedure, a patch is placed on the eye to protect it until the anaesthesia wears off.

Topical

This means eye drops. Instead of a needle, freezing drops are used. Because you still have the ability to move the eye, your surgeon may instruct you where to look. This form of anaesthesia is reserved for use with phacoemulsification and intravenous sedation is often used here as well. Immediately after the operation, vision is usually good, sometimes even 20/20. Often, no patch is required.

Although topical anaesthesia is becoming more and more popular, it may not be for everyone. Ideally, it should be the choice of a cooperative, relaxed patient and a surgeon who is comfortable and experienced in this technique.

SELECTION OF THE INTRAOCULAR LENS

At the risk of oversimplifying things, the most important thing in a cataract extraction is to take out the cloudy crystalline lens. The most important thing in a refractive lensectomy is to implant an intraocular lens of the correct power and that is not as easy as you may think.

There are several factors which are used to select the intraocular lens power.

Axial length

The length of the eye is important because it corresponds to the position of the retina. In a myope, the axial length is longer than normal, and the retina is farther away from the cornea. Therefore, any calculation of IOL power requires an accurate axial length measurement. It would be fairly uncomfortable, not to mention a bit self-defeating, to have a ruler jabbed into the eye. Instead, an ultrasound machine, or *A-Scan*, is used to determine the axial length.

Keratometry

The power of the cornea is responsible for most of the eye's refraction, so it is important to know this value. Through the use of a keratometer, which quantifies light reflections from the cornea, the diopteric power of the cornea can be measured.

The intraocular lens

The location and composition of the implant play a role in the selection of the appropriate power.

The desired refraction

Believe it or not, 20/20 is not always the best answer. If you were given the choice of one particular distance where things would be the most clear, what would you choose? Remember, as soon as your crystalline lens is removed, your accommodation is lost. When given the choice, many people elect to see perfectly clear at a distance and to use reading glasses for near vision. Others, however, prefer to be naturally focused for up close vision, and to wear distance glasses. In the case of a bilateral operation, a wise goal is to have one eye with a planned refraction of plano. The second eye can then be slightly myopic, perhaps -1 D. This difference is small enough that most people do not even notice it. It does, however, improve the range of binocular visual acuity. This approach is similar to the planned monovision in other refractive procedures.

Once all of these numbers have been decided upon, they are entered into a computer. The IOL power is calculated and offered to the surgeon. Special considerations or surgeon experience may impact that selection at this time, but usually before an instrument touches the eye, the IOL has been chosen.

Post-operative Course

The first day

The immediate post-operative course depends largely on the type of anaesthesia which was used. Following topical anaesthesia, your eye is open and vision may be very good from the moment your operation ends. Your eye may be slightly uncomfortable, but pain is infrequent. Pain with associated nausea and vomiting may be an indication that the IOP is elevated. Eye drops, usually antibiotics and steroids, and sometimes pills, are prescribed. Your follow-up appointment is usually the day following surgery.

If you were given an injection of anaesthetic, the first day is somewhat different. The vision is impaired because of the anaesthesia, but that doesn't matter because your eye is patched. Your eye is numb post-operatively and the eyelid is not functioning properly. The patch is designed to protect your eye from injury and it usually remains on until the first post-operative visit.

The first visit is important. Not only does it give your surgeon an opportunity to check for high IOP or infection, but also to check your vision. If the preliminary refraction reveals a large under or over-correction, replacement of the IOL may be considered.

The first week

As post-operative inflammation and corneal swelling subside, your vision gradually improves. Some people take a little while to become accustomed to the change in vision. For instance, colors may appear slightly different after a lens extraction. Any irritation which was present in the first couple of days also usually resolves. You continue to take the eye drops for the entire week and a post-operative visit is often scheduled around the one week mark.

The first month

The majority of the healing takes place during the first month. The eye is comfortable and vision is good. Antibiotic eye drops are usually stopped at the seven to ten days post-operatively, while the steroid drops are gradually reduced throughout the month. A post-operative visit may be scheduled for a few weeks after the surgery. If sutures were placed, they may be removed at this time. Because of continued healing, the final refraction doesn't stabilize for a few weeks. It is usually advisable to wait a little while before getting a prescription for reading glasses. There is no point in changing the glasses repeatedly as the eye heals.

The first year

The first year should be uneventful. Regardless, both you and your surgeon should be aware of the possibility of late complications (which will be described later) such as retinal detachment, cystoid macular edema, and chronic infection. In addition, posterior capsule opacification may develop. Any visual change or pain should be reported to your eye doctor.

Results

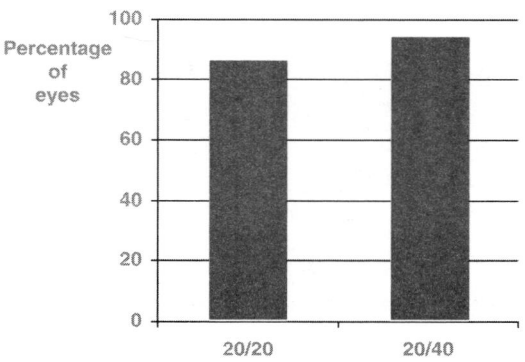

Lensectomy
Surgical Results for Myopia
(Pre-operative Refraction -10.00 to -25.00 D)

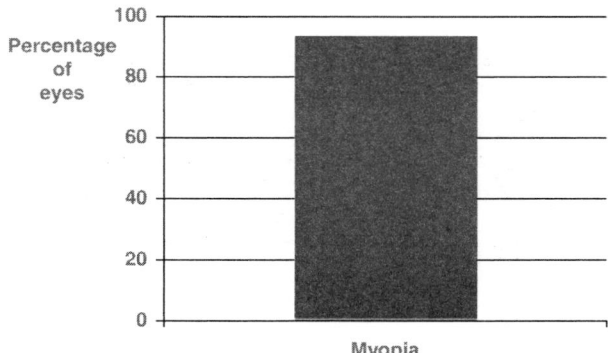

Lensectomy
Surgical Results
Within ± 1.00 D of Intended Correction

COMPLICATIONS

Undercorrection/Overcorrection

A post-operative result of plano may not always be achieved.

> Why? The power of the implant is derived from a complex formula based on several variables (including an estimate of the exact final position of the implant after the eye has healed completely). The slightest inaccuracy may result in a post-operative refractive error.

> Numbers: With high myopia or hyperopia, significant undercorrection or overcorrection may be seen in approximately 10% of eyes. This number decreases when lower refractive errors are treated.

> Treatment: Conservative options include glasses and contacts. If the post-operative refractive error is significant, removal and replacement of the IOL may be warranted. This procedure, however, is not without risks.

> Prognosis: The visual prognosis is excellent.

Infection

Ocular infections are a serious post-operative complication.

> Why? Any time the contents of the eye are exposed to the outside world, there is the chance of an infection. In contrast to the post-operative PRK situation, here the infection may be *inside* the eye. Just as with a globe perforation in RK, therefore, endophthalmitis is a consideration.

> Numbers: The chance of developing a post-operative intraocular infection is less than 0.1% (one in a thousand). If such a problem occurs, it is usually seen in the first week.

> Treatment: Prevention of endophthalmitis is, of course,

paramount. Sterile techniques and antibiotics are surgical requirements. If this complication does occur, timely intervention is necessary. The mainstay of treatment is antibiotics, and further surgery may be required.

Prognosis: Although it is possible to lose an eye from endophthalmitis, with treatment this happens uncommonly. Some loss of visual acuity is the usual end result.

Hemorrhage

Intraocular bleeding may have serious consequences.

Why? Once an eye is exposed to the outside world, the sudden change in pressure may cause blood vessels inside the eye to bleed.

Numbers: With current techniques, it is very rare (less than one in a thousand) to encounter a hemorrhage during a lensectomy.

Treatment: If a significant hemorrhage is detected, the surgeon must abort the procedure and suture the wound. Usually, the hemorrhage resolves without damage. Depending on the extent of the hemorrhage, further surgery may be necessary.

Prognosis: Visual acuity is usually not decreased significantly. However, in the event of a severe hemorrage, the eye may be lost.

Posterior Capsule Opacification (PCO)

This is more of a side effect than a complication. It is a predictable and treatable result of surgery.

Why? The posterior lens capsule which is left in the eye to support the PCIOL, can turn cloudy. Depending on the degree of opacification, vision can be affected.

Numbers: PCO occurs in about 25% of eyes following a lensectomy. The time interval is variable, ranging from weeks to years. Typically, people who see very well after surgery begin to notice a decline in their vision. Glare, halos and night vision disturbances are often reported. It is almost as if the cataract has returned. Another name for PCO is *secondary cataract.*

Treatment: The decision depends on the extent of PCO. Mild, visually insignificant opacification may be simply observed. If vision is adversely affected, a YAG laser (different from the excimer laser) may be used to make a hole, a *capsulotomy,* in this cloudy membrane.

Prognosis: A capsulotomy is usually successful in restoring vision. Potential infrequent complications of this treatment include increased IOP, increased chance of retinal detachment, and the possibility of intraocular inflammation.

Astigmatism

Removal of the crystalline lens can expose previously compensated corneal astigmatism

Why? The total astigmatism of an eye is comprised of the corneal astigmatism and the residual (lens) astigmatism. If the corneal astigmatism is +1 D and the residual astigmatism is -1 D, the net pre-operative astigmatism is zero. After the lens is removed, the corneal astigmatism is exposed, the uncorrected visual acuity may be reduced.

Numbers: This phenomenon is predictable and should be anticipated based on pre-operative testing.

Treatment: Awareness of this potential effect is important in the selection of appropriate surgical candidates. Post-operative astigmatism may be treated with conservative measures such as glasses and contacts, or surgical methods.

Prognosis: Best-corrected visual acuity is not impaired and uncorrected vision may improve with treatment.

Retinal Detachment

Lensectomy puts the eye at an increased risk of developing a retinal detachment.

Why? Several factors are involved, including retinal tears or holes, and changes in the vitreous gel.

Numbers: The numbers depend on several factors, including the degree of refractive error. High myopes, for example, have an increased chance of developing a retinal detachment. The presence of predisposing retinal abnormalities also increases the chance. In general, the risk is on the order of 1% or less. The majority of detachments happen within the first year of surgery.

Treatment: Many potential retinal detachments may be prevented by careful pre-operative management. Identification and treatment of predisposing tears is vital. Also, patient education is important in early recognition. Symptoms such as floaters, flashing lights, or a curtain appearing across the visual field, should be reported immediately. Treatment of a retinal detachment involves specialized surgery.

Prognosis: Often there is some loss of visual acuity following retinal detachment, even after successful surgical repair. About half of eyes with a treated retinal detachment will end up with vision worse than 20/50. A number of factors are involved, including the extent and duration of the detachment, so time is a relevant concern.

Cystoid Macular Edema (CME)

Swelling of the retina may cause a decrease in vision.

Why? There may be identifiable reasons such as persistent intraocular inflammation. Conversely, CME can occur out of the blue.

<u>Numbers:</u> With newer techniques, this becomes a visually significant problem in less than 1% of eyes. It usually appears early in the post-operative period and tends to resolve spontaneously.

<u>Treatment:</u> In order to diagnose CME, a special test may be performed. A fluorescein angiogram consists of a dye injection into a vein, followed by sequential retinal photographs. Many eyes with CME improve by themselves. If there are specific reasons predisposing to CME, they should be treated. In addition, eye drops have demonstrated some usefulness.

Others

In addition to the serious complications listed above, there are a few other problems which may be seen following a lensectomy. Light sensitivity, glare, double vision, dry eyes, irritation, eyelid swelling, and ptosis may occur. These problems are usually infrequent, mild, or transient and do not often cause significant problems.

MULTIFOCAL IOLS

If there can be multifocal glasses, why can't there by multifocal IOLs? The good news is that they do exist, they have been used for years, and there are people who are ecstatic to have them. Imagine having a cataract removed and being able to see near and far without any glasses. For some people, these magical multifocal IOLs represent the fountain of youth. Others see things a little differently. Although they allow you to get away without glasses, multifocal IOLs have been known to compromise your vision. Not a lot, usually, and not noticeably in everybody. Still, suppose you are given a choice of crystal clear vision for distance, except that you need reading glasses. The alternative is fairly good near and distance vision without glasses. Which way would you go? It is an individual choice, but most people tend to choose the former. A word of hope. Things are improving. It may be just a matter of time until you can choose the best of both worlds.

Summary

Advantages
- Predictable results
- Visual improvement quicker than PRK
- Minimal pain
- Short-term eye drops
- Effective in myopia and hyperopia
- No regression effect

Disadvantages
- Loss of accommodation
- Serious risks of intraocular surgery
- Opacification of posterior capsule

Best in...

<u>Significant cataract and refractive error:</u> If you have a significant cataract and refractive error, then the most difficult decision is whether or not to have surgery. If the answer is yes, then the type of surgery is not really an issue. Corneal procedures alone, including RK and PRK, would not address the cataract. Although they may improve uncorrected vision, the best-corrected vision would remain poor. Removal of the cataract along with the implant of an appropriate intraocular lens is probably the best solution. Ideally, this will improve both the best-corrected and uncorrected vision. If significant astigmatism is also present, then this can be addressed at the time of surgery.

<u>Over fifty with early cataracts</u>: In this situation, it may be worth considering a lensectomy. Chances are that your cataracts will progress and when that happens, the effect of the corneal surgery will be negated. If you're going to need a cataract extraction in the not too distant future, one argument says might as well do it now.

THE SURGICAL TREATMENT OF OTHER REFRACTIVE ERRORS

9

ASTIGMATISM

Eyes with astigmatism are a different ball game entirely. In general, there are two options.

IGNORE THE ASTIGMATISM

In eyes with a small amount of astigmatism (less than 1 D) and no associated myopia or hyperopia, this is an option. The astigmatism is probably not contributing greatly to a decrease in the vision, and if you are happy, why rock the boat?

TREAT THE ASTIGMATISM

There are several ways of treating the astigmatism:

Astigmatic Keratotomy (AK)

AK is to astigmatism what RK is to myopia. Strategically placed cuts in the cornea allow it to assume a different shape. Whereas in RK the goal is to flatten the cornea in all directions, in AK the plan is more precise. The idea is to flatten the cornea in a specific meridian.

> How? AK is performed under topical anaesthesia. A multitude of corneal incision types have been used throughout the years, but the principle remains the same. One of the most popular approaches uses *arcuate* incisions to achieve the corneal flattening.

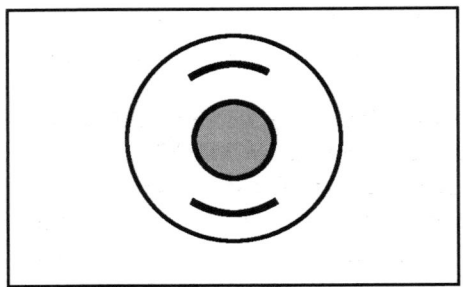

Results: AK is effective in reducing the amount of astigmatism.

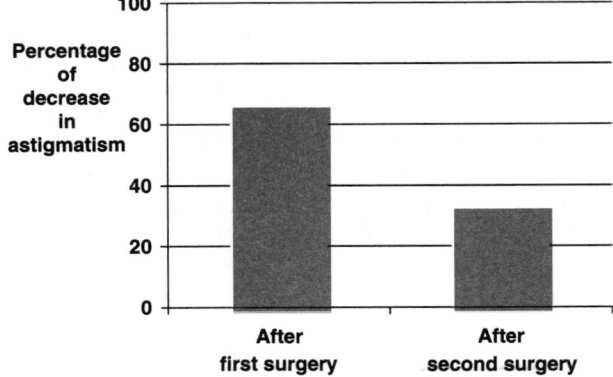

AK
Surgical Results
(1.00 to 6.00 D of Astigmatism Pre-operatively)

PRK

Thirty percent of patients who are myopic also have significant astigmatism. For this reason, researchers have turned their attention to the use of the excimer laser in the treatment of astigmatism.

How? In pure myopes, the laser is directed toward the cornea in a uniform fashion. The goal is to apply the same ablative power to the entire surface, which results in a uniform change of refraction. In astigmatic eyes, the goal is different. In order to affect the cylindrical power of the cornea, the power must be applied in a nonuniform fashion. Certain areas of the cornea are ablated more than others. This is required to turn the astigmatic football into a spherical basketball (see Chapter 3).

The lasers themselves have incorporated devices which enable the surgeon to perform these *toric* ablations. It is just a matter of programming the laser with the pertinent information. The only appreciable difference in the patient's experience is a few extra seconds of laser time. Any astigmatic correction must be performed in addition to, not instead of, the myopic or hyperopic correction.

Results: Anytime astigmatism joins the picture, everything becomes a little more complicated. Instead of dealing with a simple myopic prescription, such as -3 D, two other numbers enter the equation. The amount and axis of the correcting cylinder must be determined and treated. The results, not surprisingly, are less impressive than in simple myopia. Everything depends on degree. Mild myopes usually have mild astigmatism, and the results of PRK are very good. As the extent of myopia increases, often times so does the astigmatism. The corresponding results suffer somewhat. The bottom line is that astigmatism reduces the chance of achieving 20/20 uncorrected vision post-operatively. And the greater the astigmatism, the lower the chance.

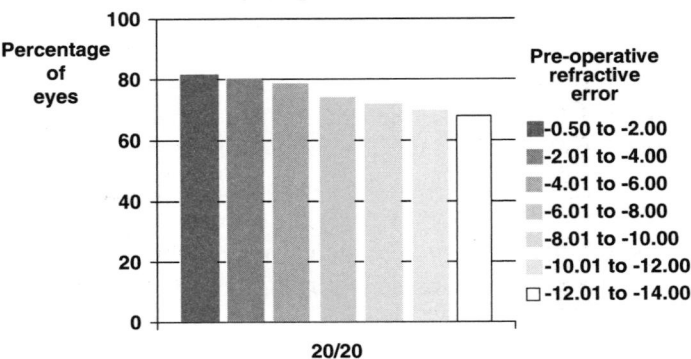

PRK
Surgical Results for Myopia <u>with</u> Astigmatism > 1.00 D
After First Procedure

Post-operative uncorrected visual acuity

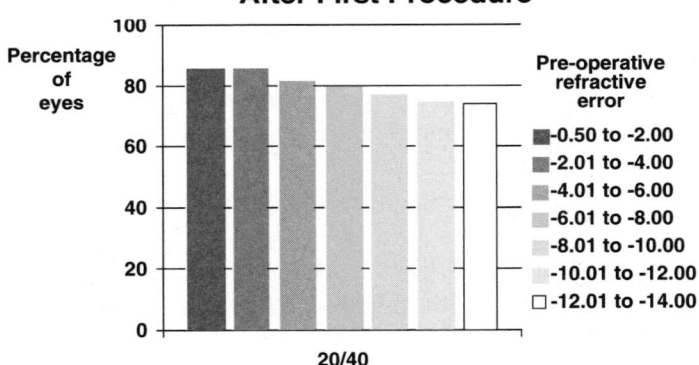

PRK
Surgical Results for Myopia <u>with</u> Astigmatism > 1.00 D
After First Procedure

Post-operative uncorrected visual acuity

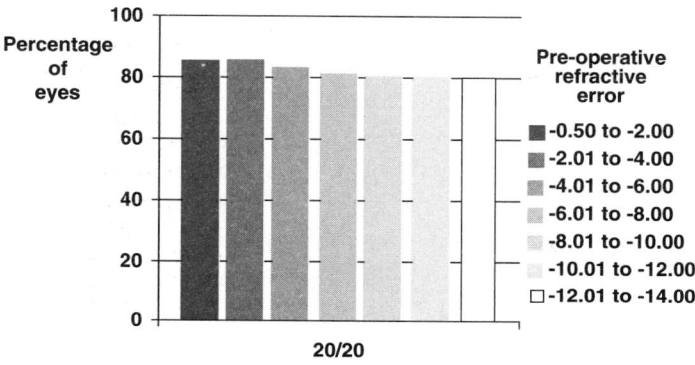

PRK
Surgical Results for Myopia <u>with</u> Astigmatism > 1.00 D
After All Procedures

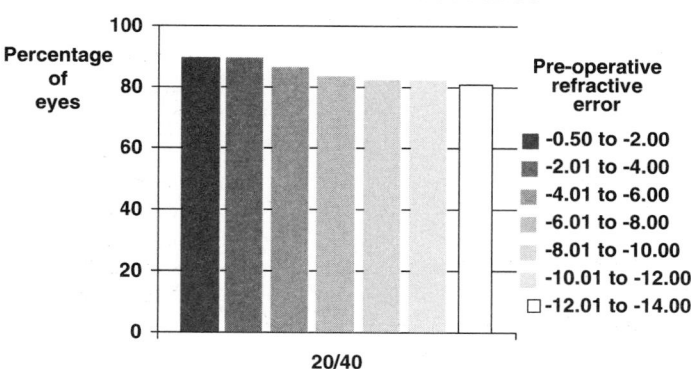

PRK
Surgical Results for Myopia <u>with</u> Astigmatism > 1.00 D
After All Procedures

LASIK

Astigmatism may be corrected with LASIK by performing toric laser ablations.

How? When performed in conjunction with a myopic or hyperopic LASIK, as is most often the case, a few extra seconds will do the trick. The flap is raised and the pre-programmed laser carves a cylindrical correction into the stromal bed.

Results: As with PRK, the success of myopic LASIK is slightly reduced when astigmatism is present. The good news is that the results are still fairly impressive, especially in eyes with high astigmatism.

LASIK
Surgical Results for Myopia <u>with</u> Astigmatism > 1.00 D
After First Procedure

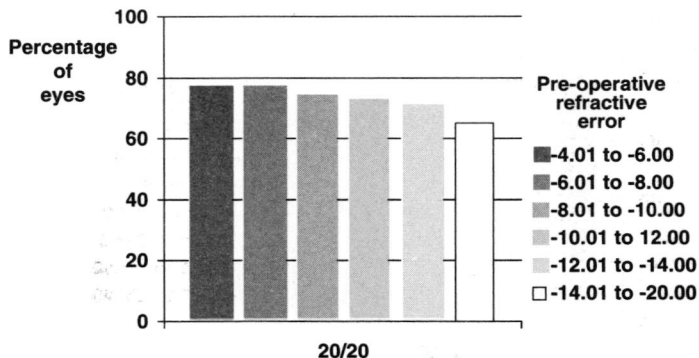

Post-operative uncorrected visual acuity

LASIK
Surgical Results for Myopia <u>with</u> Astigmatism > 1.00 D
After First Procedure

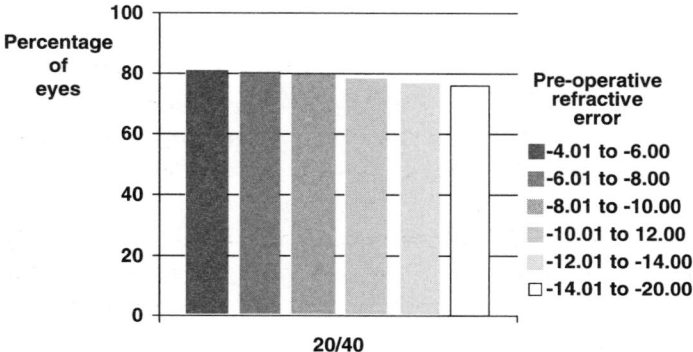

Percentage of eyes

Pre-operative refractive error

■ -4.01 to -6.00
■ -6.01 to -8.00
■ -8.01 to -10.00
□ -10.01 to 12.00
□ -12.01 to -14.00
□ -14.01 to -20.00

20/40

Post-operative uncorrected visual acuity

LASIK
Surgical Results for Myopia <u>with</u> Astigmatism > 1.00 D
After All Procedures

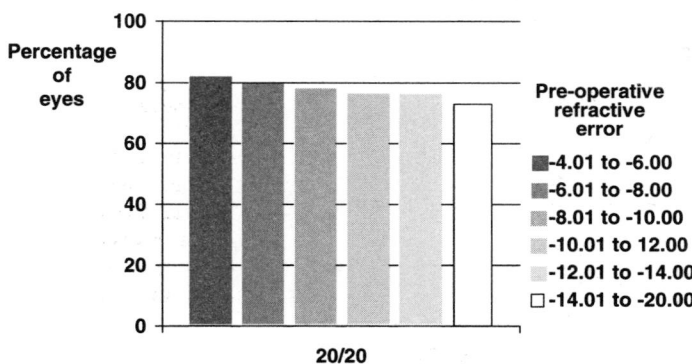

Percentage of eyes

Pre-operative refractive error

■ -4.01 to -6.00
■ -6.01 to -8.00
■ -8.01 to -10.00
□ -10.01 to 12.00
□ -12.01 to -14.00
□ -14.01 to -20.00

20/20

Post-operative uncorrected visual acuity

LASIK
Surgical Results for Myopia <u>with</u> Astigmatism > 1.00 D
After All Procedures

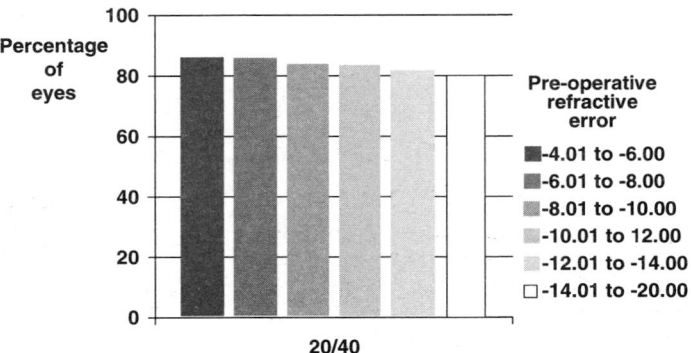

Post-operative uncorrected visual acuity

Astigmatism and refractive lensectomy

If there is significant astigmatism, it can be addressed at the time of the surgery. This can be done by manipulating the nature and location of the cataract incision, or alternatively by performing the appropriate corneal incisions. Following surgery, persistent significant astigmatism may be treatable with excimer laser techniques or AK.

SUMMARY

Predictability

AK has been around for a long time. Surgeons who have been performing the procedure for years have great confidence in this procedure. Not only is it simple, safe, and effective, it is also predictable. There is considerable intersurgeon variability, but the same doctor performing the same exact surgery, has a pretty good idea how much correction their procedure will create. Therefore, your surgeon should be confident that his or her 2 mm incision is just what the doctor ordered.

In PRK, the ability to hit the refractive target may be less when astigmatism enters the scene. For several reasons, the accuracy of the results is not as consistent. However, the outcome is pretty good and improving every day. Still, if you lived in a world where you had to have PRK and where you could pick your refractive error, it would be smart not to choose any astigmatism.

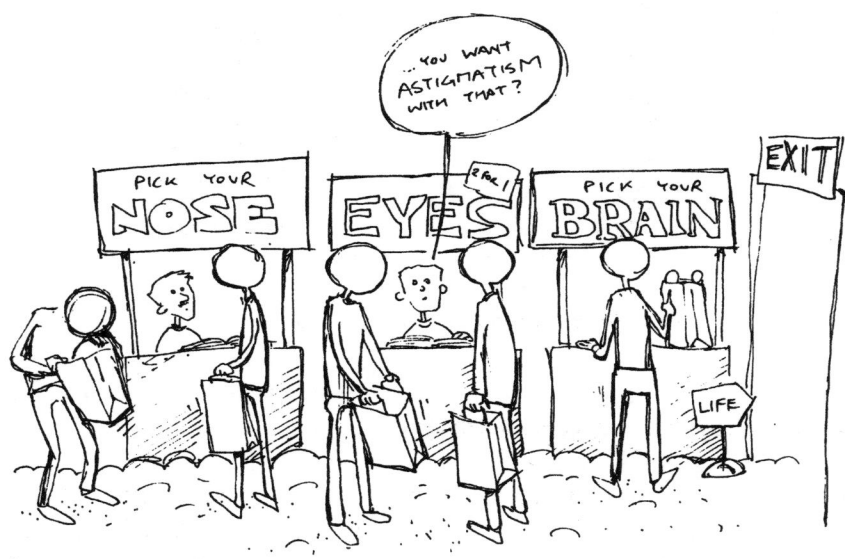

When considering an eye with significant myopic astigmatism, LASIK offers greater predictability than PRK. This is due, in large part, to the minimal myopic regression seen in LASIK. Instead of having to putt with a huge left to right break, you can aim for the centre of the cup.

Track record

There are people walking around who had AK performed ten years ago. It should be somewhat reassuring to know that this procedure has been around so long. The track record for PRK is inferior. Not in quality, but in length. There is more long-term data on AK, but the initial trends of astigmatic PRK are good. LASIK is the new kid on the astigmatic block. Although early results of LASIK are encouraging, long-term stability and efficacy have yet to be established.

Precision

AK is low-tech, and depending on your views of technology, that may be a plus. The less complicated a machine, the less chance of technological error. Microchips which do not exist cannot malfunction. AK is extremely precise. Still, a laser beam is *much* more precise than the hands of the best surgeon in the world. Just by looking at the laser grooves carved on a hair, it is impossible to refute that simple fact. It is no contest. Does the precision of a surgical instrument translate to a superior clinical outcome? That is the real question. A state-of-the-art computer is useless if you don't know how to work the mouse. The results indicate that AK may be comparable to the laser techniques. The debate continues.

Safety

Safety is a relative term, especially when knives and lasers are brought into contact with an eye. In AK, the cornea is being cut to depths of 90% thickness. Operative complications can result. Furthermore, trauma to the post-operative eye can result in devastating consequences. Of course these are simply worst-case scenario considerations. But they are worth considering. When contrasted to AK, the structural integrity of the eye is much less compromised with PRK. Even LASIK cuts only at 20% to 30% of corneal thickness. Consequently, the laser techniques may leave the eye less vulnerable to minor trauma.

Hyperopic and myopic astigmatism

When a combination of refractive errors coexist, AK will only solve the problem of astigmatism. In order to address the other problems, AK must be supplemented by a further procedure such as RK. PRK and LASIK can do with a few extra seconds what a blade can do with a few extra incisions. The advantage of the laser techniques is that hyperopic astigmatism may be treated.

High astigmatism

High astigmatism responds well to PRK. Percentage-wise, even better than low astigmatism. An 80% reduction in your high astigmatism will take you from 5 D to 1 D. Conversely, a fifty percent drop in your low 1 D astigmatism will leave you with 0.5 D. Even if the results aren't perfect, PRK for high astigmatism may be rewarding.

Still, the greater the astigmatism, the greater chance of problems. Undercorrection and overcorrection occur at an increased frequency with all techniques. AK requires more longer and deeper incisions which may result in halos, glare, and fluctuating vision. Using PRK to treat high astigmatism increases the incidence of corneal haze. The preliminary results of LASIK suggest that it may be the treatment of choice in high astigmatism, but it is still early in the game.

Cost

Laser procedures are invariably more expensive than the incisional techniques.

10

HYPEROPIA
AND PRESBYOPIA

For the treatment of myopia, there are several reasonable treatment options. For hyperopia, the answer is not so clear cut.

When you talk about surgically treating hyperopia, the issue of presbyopia goes hand in hand. If someone is fifty years old and has a refractive error of plano in each eye, they can probably see 20/20 in the distance. For reading, however, they need glasses. Their myopic friends, conversely, can read without glasses. The ideal situation would be if one eye were plano and the other eye were slightly myopic. This is *monovision,* which was discussed in Chapter 4. Moving from plano to -1 D is not that different than moving from +1 D to plano. The treatment modalities are the same, and for this reason, the treatment of presbyopia is considered analogous to that of hyperopia.

INTRAOCULAR SURGERY

Cataract extraction or refractive lensectomy are reasonable methods of treating hyperopia. The risks and benefits are the same (or less than) as for myopic lensectomy and are outlined in Chapter 8. In addition, phakic IOL's (see Chapter 11) may have a role to play in hyperopia down the road.

Results

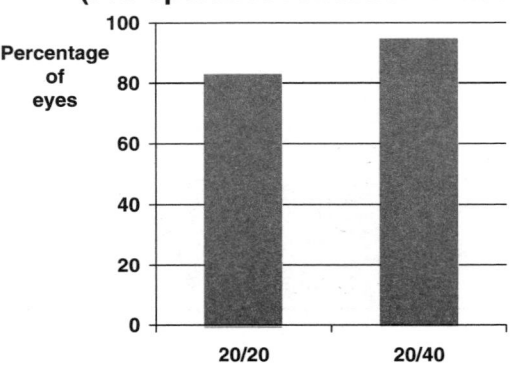

Lensectomy
Surgical Results for Hyperopia
(Pre-operative refraction + 4.00 to +10.00 D)

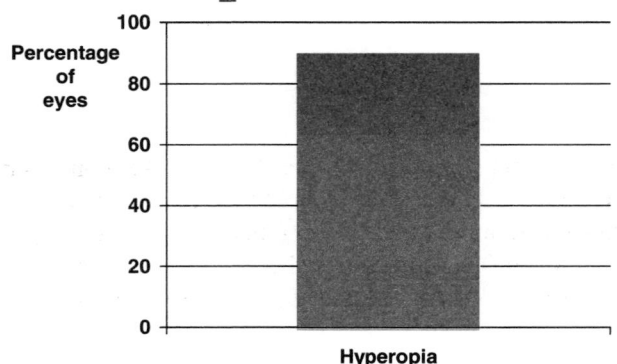

Lensectomy
Surgical Results
Within ± 1.00 D of Intended Correction

Incisional Surgery

Hexagonal Keratotomy

If one can make cuts in a myopic cornea which allow it to flatten, as in RK, it is conceivable that strategically placed incisions may encourage a hyperopic cornea to steepen. The opposite of RK, as it turns out, is a procedure known as *hexagonal keratotomy* (HK). As the name suggests, the cuts form a six-sided geometric shape on the cornea.

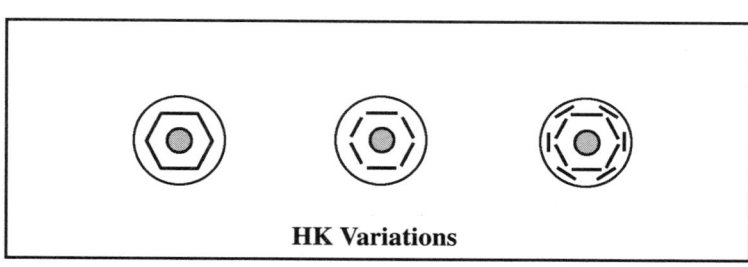

HK Variations

The procedure: HK has been employed in the treatment of low hyperopia (<6 D). Similar to RK, this operation is performed under topical anaesthesia with a diamond knife.

Complications: The inherent risks of incisional surgery are common to both procedures. The complication profile of HK is similar to that of RK and includes glare, fluctuating vision, irregular astigmatism, perforation, infection, corneal weakness.

ALK

Hyperopic ALK differs from the myopic version. The microkeratome performs its pass at a greater depth, at about 60% corneal thickness. When the flap is created, the thin stromal bed bulges under the influence of intraocular pressure. When the flap is repositioned, it conforms to the bulge, creating a steeper cornea. There is no need to excise any corneal tissue. The first pass of the microkeratome is the only pass.

The procedure: With the exception that there is no excision of corneal tissue, hyperopic ALK is performed similarly to myopic ALK. The amount of steepening is dependent on the diameter of the flap.

Complications: All of the risks inherent to ALK apply in the hyperopic version as well. In addition, there is the added problem of corneal weakening, which, in its severe state, can require a corneal transplant.

LASER TECHNIQUES

Holmium-YAG Laser Thermal Keratoplasty (LTK)

A different kind of laser has also been used in the treatment of hyperopia. The holmium:YAG laser differs from the excimer in that it produces heat. When directed at the cornea, this laser causes collagen fibres to shrink, thereby altering the curvature of the cornea. The FDA has not yet approved the laser for LTK.

The Procedure: The pre-operative testing and preparation follow the same protocol as other refractive procedures. The variables which must be addressed prior to surgery are the laser spot size, pattern, energy, and total number.

Under topical anaesthesia, the eye is centred under the laser aiming beam. The

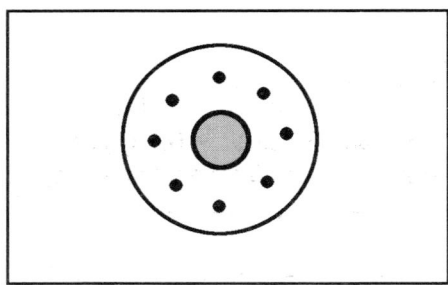

laser is then fired for a total of two to four seconds. Antibiotic drops are placed in the eye and you are on your way.

Complications: Mild pain, light sensitivity, and tearing are reported by about half of the patients immediately post-operatively. By three days after the operation, these symptoms usually disappear. Hyperopic regression is common and has been called the Achilles' heel of LTK. The eye drifts back toward its original refractive error, months after the surgery. Irregular astigmatism may also be induced by this procedure, which can result in a decrease in best corrected vision.

Results:

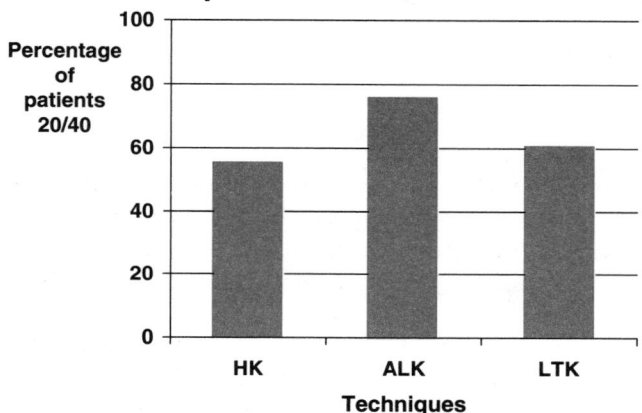

HK, ALK, LTK
Surgical Results for Hyperopia
Post-operative Uncorrected Visual Acuity

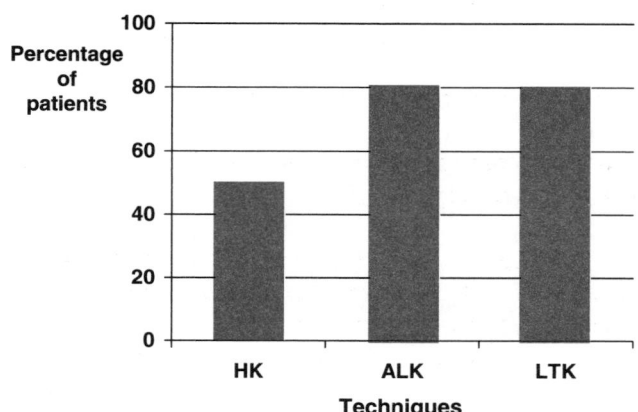

HK, ALK, LTK
Surgical Results for Hyperopia
Within $\pm$ 1.00 D Intended Correction

HK, ALK, LTK
Surgical Results for Hyperopia
Loss of ≥ 2 lines of Best Corrected Visual Acuity

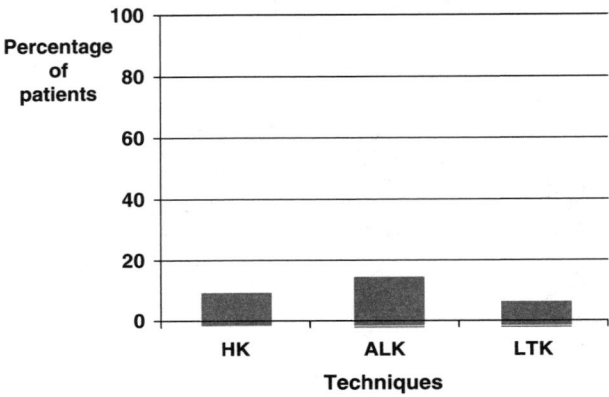

PRK

PRK can be used to steepen the cornea in the treatment of hyperopia. In contrast to myopic PRK, here the laser ablates more in the peripheral cornea than the central part. The deepest sculpting occurs in a ring pattern, with the central visual axis being relatively spared. This results in a steepening of the central cornea, thereby reducing the hyperopia.

The Procedure: PRK is being used for low and moderate levels of hyperopia (<5-6 D) It is performed in a similar fashion to myopic PRK. The laser is applied to a larger diameter treatment zone, around 9 mm, with the centre remaining relatively spared. The post-operative course is similar to that of myopic PRK.

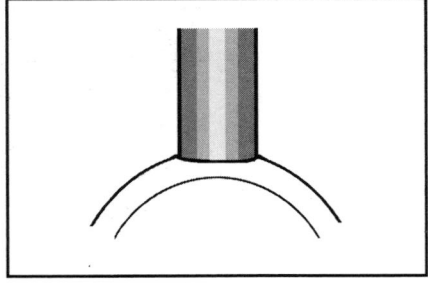

Results:

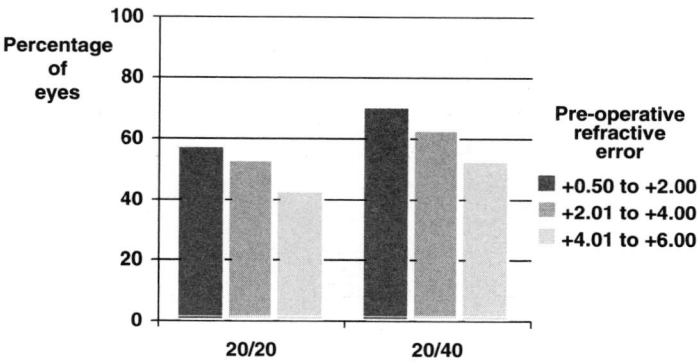

PRK
Surgical Results for Hyperopia
After First Procedure

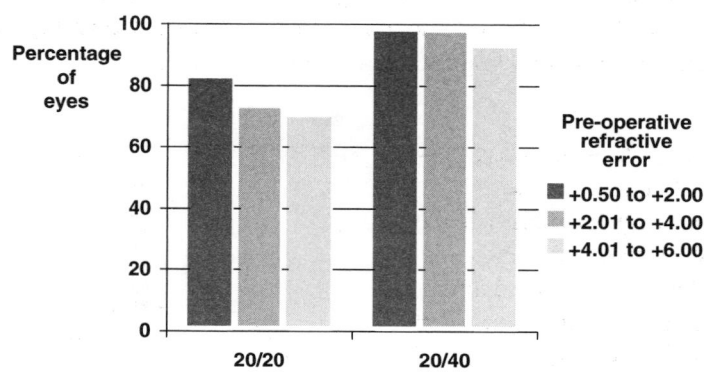

PRK
Surgical Results for Hyperopia
After All Procedures

PRK
Surgical Results for Hyperopia
Within ± 1.00 D of Intended Correction

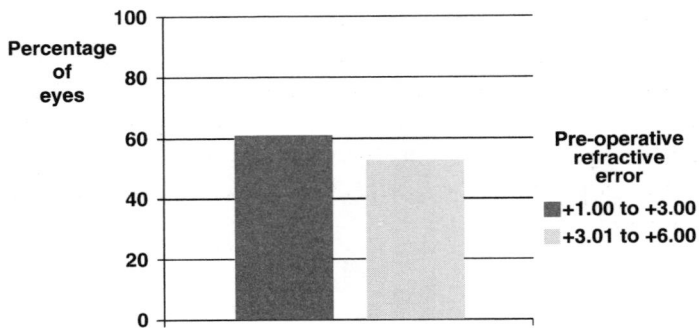

PRK
Surgical Results for Hyperopia
Number of Treatments per Eye

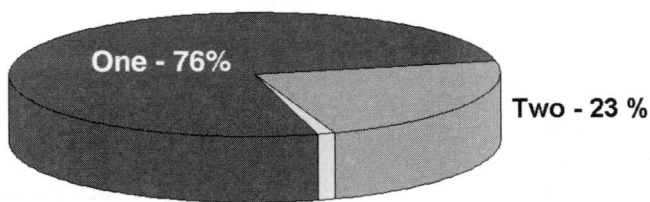

Complications: The complications seen in myopic PRK (Chapter 5) also occur in hyperopic PRK. Corneal haze, however, is less of a concern. Although it is observed commonly, the haze is typically more pronounced in a peripheral ring than it is centrally. This corresponds to the zone where the laser ablation was the deepest. The central cornea is typically spared of significant haze. Consequently, visual acuity is not usually affected. Because of the large diameter treatment zone, epithelialization of the cornea becomes more of a problem. In general, it takes a little longer, which increases the morbidity and risks associated with a persistent epithelial defect. Another difference involves the regression effect. Although seen in hyperopia as well, it tends to work in the opposite direction. The drift is toward the starting point. A pre-operative hyperope often regresses back toward hyperopia, as opposed to the myopic situation.

LASIK

The procedure: Hyperopic LASIK is similar to its myopic cousin. The difference is that the laser is focused in a ring-like fashion, with the peripheral cornea receiving more treatment than the centre. This results in a steepening of the visual axis which eliminates the hyperopia.

Results:

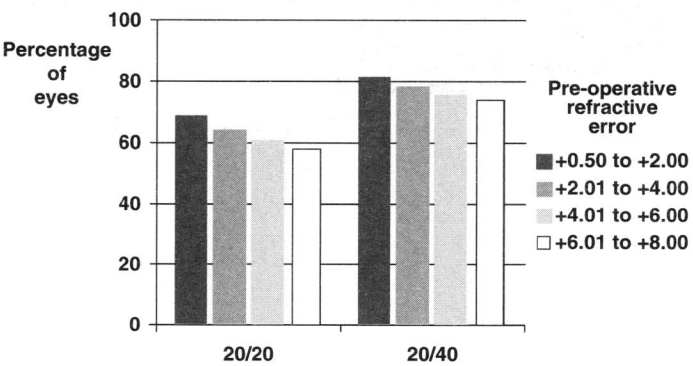

LASIK
Surgical Results for Hyperopia
After First Procedure

Percentage of eyes

Pre-operative refractive error

■ +0.50 to +2.00
▨ +2.01 to +4.00
▧ +4.01 to +6.00
☐ +6.01 to +8.00

20/20   20/40

Post-operative uncorrected visual acuity

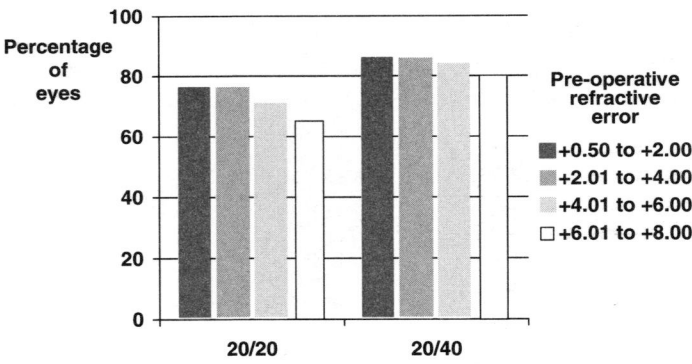

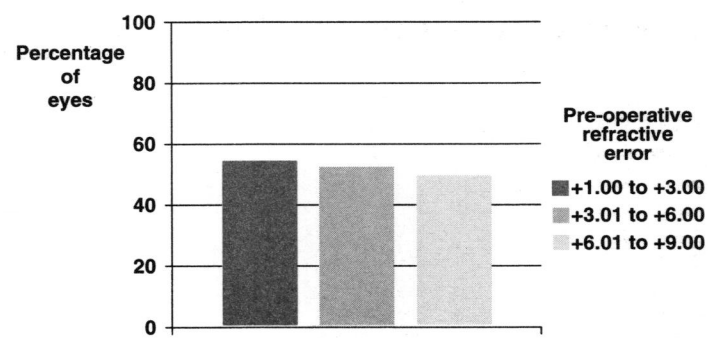

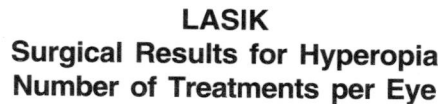

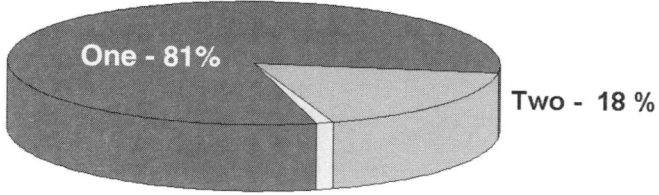

Complications: All of the risks inherent to LASIK in general (see Chapter 6) apply to this specific procedure. In addition, there is a special factor which merits consideration. When hyperopic LASIK is performed, a large diameter of the cornea is ablated to cause the necessary steepening. The effective optical zone, however, is relatively small. This may give rise to symptoms such as halos. Also, some individuals may notice a decrease in their ability to distinguish objects of low contrast.

SUMMARY

Predictability

HK is falling out of favor among ophthalmologists, partly because of its less than perfect predictability. Although LTK may be somewhat more predictable in the immediate post-operative period, regression rears its ugly head as months go by. Long-term results are less encouraging, but new studies with newer lasers are more promising, demonstrating stable results in corrections up to 2 to 3 D. ALK is somewhat less predictable. PRK and LASIK are demonstrating a high degree of predictability at low levels of hyperopia. Refractive lensectomy is among the most predictable of the hyperopic techniques, especially at higher degrees of hyperopia. With this procedure, individual variation in corneal wound healing is taken out of the picture. Instead, success depends mostly on the process of selecting the appropriate intraocular lens.

Track record

Lensectomy techniques and intraocular lenses have been around for a long time and have an enviable track record. HK has been around for a while, but it's track record may not be as good as it is long. ALK also suffers from an imperfect history. PRK, LTK, and LASIK are the new kids on the block. Long-term studies have yet to be performed and the jury is still out.

Precision

HK uses a hand held knife to do the deed. In contrast, PRK and LASIK have the theoretical advantage of laser precision. Although LTK also uses a laser, the manner of use may be less precise. The laser is employed to burn the cornea, not to sculpt it. Lensectomy performed by phacoemulsification is precise, as is the calculation of the IOL power.

Safety

This is the big factor which separates the contenders from the pretenders. The complication profile of HK is concerning. For starters, this incisional technique puts the eye at risk of traumatic rupture. Furthermore, it is a surgeon dependent procedure which, in some hands, can lead to a significant loss of best corrected vision. A one in ten chance of losing two lines of best corrected vision is frightening. This ballpark figure is also encountered in ALK, which is a technique giving way to LASIK. Post-operative corneal thinning is a real threat and a corneal transplant is about as fun as a root canal. Not to be outdone is LTK, which, in earlier incarnations anyway, caused significant irregular astigmatism resulting in a loss of best corrected vision. Lensectomy is a relatively safe procedure, but intraocular surgery automatically subjects you to the risk of a few uncommon but serious complications. PRK is not without risks, but the chance of intraocular problems developing are close to zero. The complications of PRK typically revolve around epithelial problems. LASIK is a relatively safe procedure, and the epithelial difficulties are minimal. However, the technically challenging nature of this surgery increases the chance of intraoperative complications. Furthermore, flap wrinkles and interface problems are always possibilities.

Range

All of the techniques are better for low hyperopia than high. PRK has an increased rate of complications at higher refractive errors, as does HK and ALK. LTK appears to be useful only for low hyperopia (about 2 D). LASIK and lensectomy are more useful for higher degrees of hyperopia, but suffer from less predictability at these levels. Until the other procedures evolve further, refractive lensectomy is likely the most accurate way of treating high hyperopia.

Accommodation

Refractive lensectomy is responsible for eliminating the eye's ability to accommodate. With the other techniques, accommodation is preserved.

Cost

The excimer laser techniques, RK and LASIK, are at the top of the price pyramid, with the other techniques occupying the ground floor. LTK will ultimately be cheaper than the excimer laser procedures.

Overcorrected eyes

An eye which was originally myopic, only to become hyperopic after refractive surgery, is termed overcorrected. The techniques which have been used for *primary* hyperopia, have also been applied to these overcorrected eyes. The results are imperfect and somewhat variable. HK and ALK are aggressive surgical modalities. In an eye which has already been weakened by a previous refractive procedure, these procedures may be poorly tolerated. Performing HK on an RK eye results in a design on the cornea which resembles a tie game of tic-tac-toe. The laser treatments are in their infancy, and the results of PRK and LASIK for the overcorrected population appear to be not quite as predictable as for the primary hyperopia group. Because of the fact that there is no perfect treatment for overcorrected eyes, prevention is the key. If overcorrection does result, the decision about the necessity and modality of treatment should be individualized.

Presbyopia

In order for it to make sense to pursue surgical monovision, the numbers should be good. If someone is plano and sees 20/20 in both eyes, it is inadvisable to subject them to an unpredictable or unsafe procedure. At present, the treatment modalities which are available are less than perfect. They are improving rapidly, however, and there is justified optimism for the future surgical treatment of presbyopia.

PART
FOUR

PERSPECTIVES

11

AN EYE ON THE FUTURE

If hindsight is 20/20, then foresight is in need of refractive surgery. The view into the crystal ball is somewhat murky. Still, a few predictions may be ventured.

ESTABLISHED TECHNIQUES

PRK

Third and higher generation lasers will emerge on the scene. Better hardware and more sophisticated software will result in even greater precision in laser energy delivery. In combination with the cumulative international experience, improvements in techniques, and greater understanding of tissue healing variability, more predictable results will be obtained. PRK will become more useful for higher ranges of refractive error and the FDA will approve these machines for hyperopia, astigmatism, and high myopia.

LASIK

In addition to taking advantage of improved laser technology, LASIK will benefit from advancements in microkeratomes. There are a number of new microkeratome concepts on the horizon which have the potential to reduce the risk of flap-related complications. As the complications drop, LASIK may be recommended for even low and moderate refractive errors.

ALK

As the laser techniques gain momentum, ALK will be regarded as yesterday's news. New more precise microkeratomes may help with the difficult task of turning the tide.

RK

Mini-RK will move to the forefront of myopic incisional techniques, however the improvements in laser surgery may make this a less attractive option. RK will likely continue to have some role in treatment of low levels of myopia.

HK

The risk profile and instability of HK, in conjunction with the improvements in the laser techniques, will likely render this procedure obsolete in the near future.

LTK

New generation holmium lasers have demonstrated promise for the treatment of low levels of hyperopia. Further studies will determine whether the issue of regression can be dealt with adequately.

Refractive Lensectomy

There will be less radical changes in this procedure than in the laser techniques, as cataract surgery has already benefitted from decades of development. Depending on the safety and efficacy of the laser techniques for high myopia and hyperopia, lensectomy may come to the forefront for the treatment of these conditions.

NEW PROCEDURES

There are researchers around the globe who are hard at work on alternative treatments for refractive errors. They hope that their new methods will, one day, make today's techniques obsolete. It is a long road from a brilliant idea to a consumer alternative, and there are many potholes along the way. There are, however, several promising ideas in the pipeline that may make the refractive surgery picture even more crowded and clouded.

Intrastromal Corneal Rings

The curvature of the cornea can be altered by other techniques. Currently under investigation in the U.S. are devices known as *intrastromal corneal ring segments* (ICRS). The idea was that if a ring is implanted within the substance of the cornea itself, the central visual axis becomes flatter.

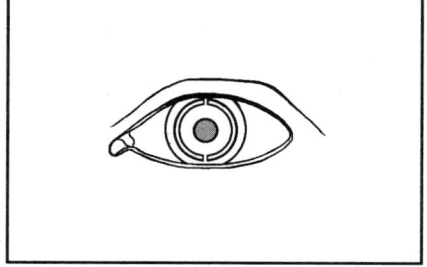

Under topical anaesthesia, an incision is made in the peripheral cornea to about two-thirds depth. A circumferential channel is dissected and the clear ring segment is then threaded around the circumference and the incision is sutured. The degree of refractive change is manipulated by altering the thickness of the ring segments.

Potential advantages of this procedure include cost (no laser required), reversibility and adjustability (the ring segments can be removed or replaced with ones of different thickness for over/undercorrections), sparing of the visual axis (no surgery is done centrally), and epithelial integrity (no scraping is necessary).

Phakic IOLs and Intraocular Contact Lenses

Let's assume you don't have a cataract. You're twenty-five years old and your crystalline lens is perfectly clear. You're just very myopic or hyperopic. Maybe it seems a little drastic to have your lens removed. After all, you would be trading the next fifteen to twenty years of perfectly good accommodation for a set of reading glasses.

Recently, somebody had a bright idea. Leave the crystalline lens in the eye *and* implant an IOL. This is called a *phakic IOL*. This way, you can change the refraction of the eye without affecting the accommodation. Sounds great in theory. In practice, it's a little tricky. Where do you put the IOL?

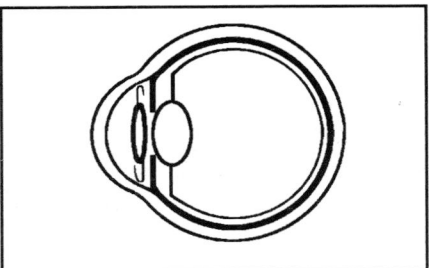

Traditionally, most implants have gone in the posterior chamber, but if the crystalline lens has now refused to vacate the spot, is there room? Some surgeons have managed to slip a PCIOL in between the iris and the crystalline lens. Others advocate ACIOLs.

Another line of thinking involves constructing a biocompatible *intraocular contact lens* (ICL). Instead of putting it on the surface of the eye, it is slipped *inside* the eye, where it rests comfortably on the crystalline lens. The ICL is a soft lens which is permeable to nutrients.

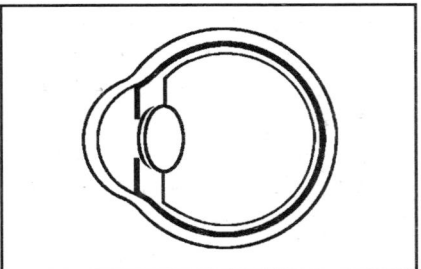

The early results of these techniques are promising, but not perfect. There have been long term studies which document the safety of IOLs, but these have been post-cataract extraction. The long-term effects of phakic IOLs and ICLs have yet to be determined, however the promise of retaining accommodative powers with an implanted lens is the driving force.

12

THE BOTTOM LINE

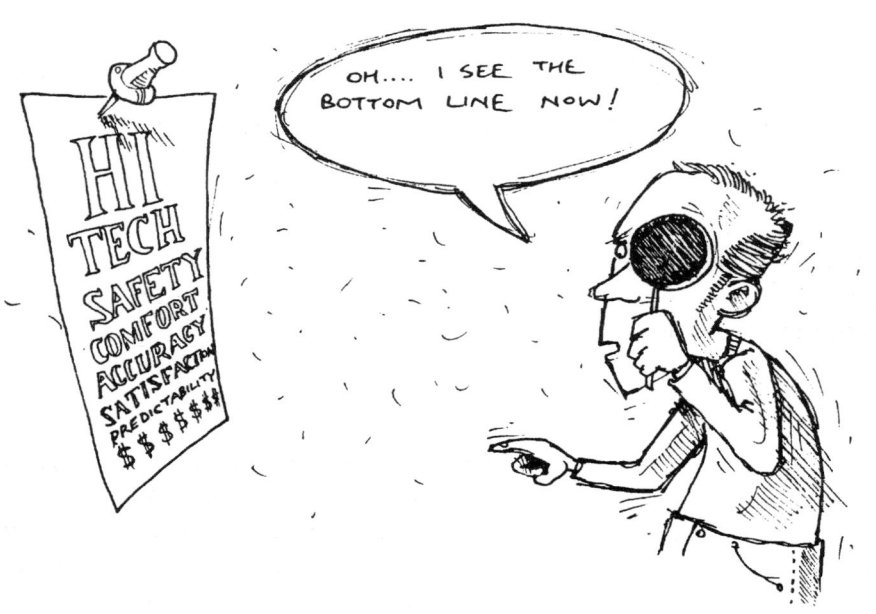

Refractive surgery is big business. Make no mistake about it. Individual doctors invest hundreds of thousands of dollars. Laser manufacturers invest millions. By the year 2000, laser eye surgery will be an $11 billion a year industry. There are laser centres which are trading as public companies on the stock exchange. This is no longer about medicine. This is about money. This is about buying and selling.

THE BUYER (*YOU*)

When you go car shopping, it is always a good idea to know a little bit about money. For starters, it is important to sit down with your bankbook and bills. Before you start picking the color of your new car, it might be nice to know if you can afford one. Or maybe a used car. Or a bicycle. Before you leave home, you should decide how much money you can afford to spend.

The same principle applies to refractive surgery. If you can spend five hundred dollars and not a penny more, so be it. See what you can get for that amount. If you're happy with the deal, do it. If not, go home and save until you can afford what you want.

THE SELLERS (*THEM*)

You already know about yourself. What you need to know about are the other guys. Before you run onto the playing field, it may be wise to learn a little bit about the stakes, the players, and the whole game of refractive surgery.

The Ophthalmologist

You have already been introduced to this player. Most often, the ophthalmologist is the one who performs the procedure. It is worthwhile noting that, by some strange coincidence, they get paid for doing so. At the risk of hitting you over the head unnecessarily, the fact is that your operation puts money in the pockets of your surgeon. Equally important, if you decide not to have the operation, the surgeon loses revenue. And if the laser is being financed by the doctor, he or she still has to pay for the laser. The bottom line is the bottom line. It is in their best financial interest to have you sign on the dotted line.

There are several possible ways for an ophthalmologist to be involved in the laser business.

A single ophthalmologist owns the laser. This is an unusual arrangement because of the costs involved.

Multiple ophthalmologists own the laser. The cost of the laser, the overhead, and the staff are shared among a group of surgeons. Each ophthalmologist is allowed use of the laser centre, perhaps on a weekly basis. Profits and losses are enjoyed and suffered by the surgeons themselves.

An ophthalmologist may have no ownership in a laser centre. Rather than refer to another surgeon, he or she may still have access to a laser. Often times there is an arrangement whereby an ophthalmologist may use the centre's facilities, with a portion of the total fee going to the laser centre.

Ophthalmologists may also refer to other surgeons for the procedure itself, in an arrangement similar to that of optometrists (described below). Rather than deal with the headache of flying the laser, they choose to do only the take-off and landing.

The Optometrist

Optometrists are big players in the world of refractive surgery, but they do not usually receive any surgical fee. Not directly anyway. Typically, optometrists have a number of patients who are potential surgical candidates. Early on, surgeons recognized that fact and vied for the favor of optometrists and their potentially lucrative referrals. Optometrists soon realized that refractive surgery was a lose-lose situation for them. Not only were they receiving no financial compensation for their referrals, but sometimes the patients never came back. A 3 D myope who became 20/20 uncorrected had no reason for a contact lens appointment. A referred patient was often a lost patient and optometrists felt that they were not receiving a fair share of the refractive surgery pie. As a result, several working relationships are found today.

Optometrists develop strategic liaisons with refractive surgeons, in a setup known as *co-management*. The details depend on the specific arrangement, but the essence is that the optometrist is involved in the care of their patient. Usually, the patient is referred back to the optometrist for post-operative care. The surgeon is the one who (in conjunction with the informed patient) makes the decision which procedure to select. After using his or her refined skills to perform the operation, the surgeon pockets his or her portion of the total fee. The remainder is billed by the referring optometrist to cover the post-operative care. Not only does this arrangement reimburse the optometrist for the follow-up care, it also ensures that the patient is not lost forever. It is important to recognize that the co-management strategy was developed for patient convenience and economic, not medical reasons.

The pros and cons of co-management are being debated in the ophthalmology community. Proponents believe that optometrists are capable professionals who are well-suited to managing their patients post-operatively. Others believe that it should be incumbent on the ophthalmologist who performs surgery to deliver the post-operative care, and that allowing the patient to go back to the referring optometrist is substandard. Vocal opponents suggest that co-management is good for the ophthalmologist, good for the optometrist, but not so good for the most important person in the equation, the patient.

Other optometrists take the matter into their own hands. They form groups which acquire ownership (or joint ownership with ophthalmologists) in laser centres. This way, there is no reason to refer patients to anyone and the entire fee remains in the family. The only problem is that optometrists, in almost every jurisdiction, cannot perform surgery. This problem is solved by hiring ophthalmologists who, for a fee, perform the procedure. With joint ownership, the ophthalmologist partners perform the surgery.

Some optometrists hope to eventually perform the procedure themselves. The numbers are still small and things are evolving as optometrists continue to lobby for permission to perform laser surgery.

The bottom line is that optometrists also have a financial interest in your decision.

The Laser Manufacturers

The companies who make the lasers have a huge stake in your decision. If you choose not to have the procedure, or if you choose RK over the excimer, they will be directly affected. Because many of the large companies are aware of the potential market for laser eye surgery, there is a great deal of competition in the industry. Behind closed doors, they are vying for the affections of ophthalmologists. Our laser is better than theirs, they cry. We were here first, shout others. The competition is coming out in the open as some laser companies figure that you, the consumer, should choose your laser.

Some laser companies are taking their product directly to the consumer. They are aggressively promoting laser centres where surgery will be performed using, big surprise, their own equipment.

There are also legal battles in the refractive arena. Patents and royalties are the issue. Although things are in a state of flux, for every excimer laser procedure performed, a royalty of $250 U.S. goes to the patent holding company.

THE FDA

The big intimidating bouncer at the door, the gatekeeper to the land of laser dollars is the FDA. Their goal it is to ensure that only effective, safe drugs and equipment reach the consumer.

In order to get into the party, laser companies must demonstrate to the FDA that their lasers are safe and effective. This involves large clinical and laboratory studies, many patients, and piles of statistics. If, and only if, the FDA is satisfied, the laser receives permission for use. In order to take the laser from the idea stage to the market, millions of dollars must be invested. All of this money, plus more for profit, must ultimately be recovered from you, the consumer.

THE STAKES

A brand new state of the art laser, with leather seats and cruise control, is expensive. Depending on your specific choice, it will cost about half a million dollars. That is for a laser alone. A maintenance contract, and what good is a

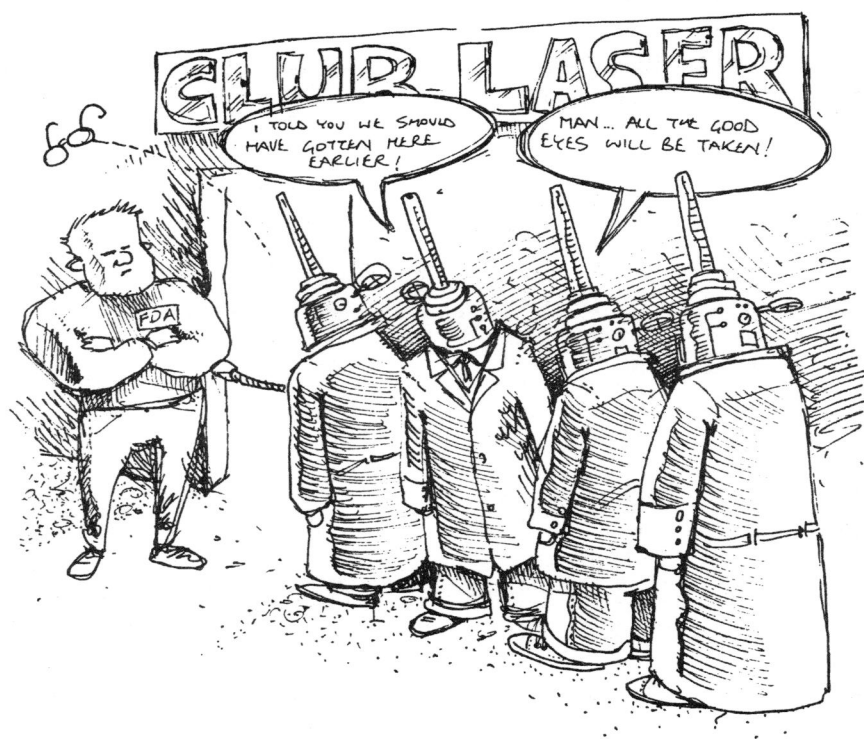

laser without proper maintenance, runs about $50,000 per year. Giving the laser a nice home will cost about as much as a nice home. Hiring and training staff adds another $100,000. The grand total is just under a million dollars, give or take. Perhaps it is becoming clearer why laser eye surgery is so expensive.

In comparison, RK sounds better and better. Chances are the Operating Room is already in place and a new home for the laser is not necessary. To perform RK, all the surgeon needs is a few instruments, a sharp knife, and a willing patient. Start-up costs are a fraction and break even numbers are small.

It doesn't matter who foots the bill for the laser centre. The bottom line is that the dollars have to be recovered. From the patient. Furthermore, if the surgeon and referring optometrist want to make even minimum wage for their time and effort, then that few bucks an hour must be added on top. And as you may have guessed, few surgeons are satisfied with minimum wage.

There are many possible arrangements. Let's take a look at a typical situation. Say the procedure costs $1600 U.S. per eye. The breakdown may be as follows:

Laser centre fee	$700
Surgeon fee	$350
Co-management fee	$300
Royalty	$250
	$1600

These figures do not represent profits, just gross income. Overhead, including marketing, reduces the net dollars even further. Some estimates suggest that for every patient who has laser surgery, as much as $200 is spent on marketing. Enhancement procedures also must be factored in. Many centres do not charge for retreatment and the surgeon's time is uncompensated.

Why do you need to know all of this? When you go car shopping, it is helpful to know the invoice price of a vehicle. If the Jeep costs the dealership $20,000, you can bargain and hold your breath and threaten to walk away, but they're not going to sell it to you for $19,000. In terms of laser eye surgery, you can bargain and hold your breath ,and wait for the price to hit $500, but you may need to change your glasses a few times in the interim.

Laser eye surgery will remain expensive. That much is clear. How expensive? Looking at the numbers, there is not a lot of flexibility there. A surgeon who gets $500 dollars for performing a cataract operation will not waste his or her time doing laser refractive surgery for much less than that. Similarly, time-consuming post-operative visits must be compensated adequately or nobody will do it. Not to be forgotten is the patent royalty which is fixed.

The big variable is the laser centres. If they become efficient, mass producing, assembly line machines, their costs will drop. They may be able to pass on savings to you. Their biggest cost, however, is the laser itself, and nobody can predict what is going to happen. Technology, as a rule, gets less expensive over time. Compare what five thousand dollars will buy on the computer market today versus five years ago. The same laser which sells for half a million dollars today may go for a fraction of that down the road. Chances are, however, that the state of the art laser five years from now will be just as expensive as today. Remember, the laser companies still have to recover all of their initial investment and compared with home computers, far fewer lasers are needed. In five years, are you going to want to save a few hundred dollars to have eye surgery with an obsolete laser?

It is possible that competition will reduce the prices for laser eye surgery. For the reasons outlined above, it seems unlikely that there will be any drastic cuts in the fee for laser eye surgery in the immediate future.

That's not to say that there aren't bargains out there. In particular, some laser centres may offer an incentive for booking both eyes. Others have borrowed from the world of automobile sales and offer their own financing. Just as with any major purchase, it doesn't hurt to do some comparison shopping. A word of caution. Dollars should be only one factor in your decision making process because on occasion, you get what you pay for.

THE COST OF NOT HAVING REFRACTIVE SURGERY

Unless you plan to take up squinting as a full time hobby, you are going to need some help, whether or not you choose to have refractive surgery. Glasses and contact lenses are not free. In order to assess the economic value of refractive surgery, it may be useful compare it to the alternatives. Let's do the math.

Assume you're a 25 year old, -4 D myope with no astigmatism. If you have refractive surgery today, you will still need reading glasses at age 45. That gives you 20 years of total freedom. Using ballpark figures and U.S. dollars:

Glasses:

Frames $100 + Lenses $100 = $200

Assume you change your glasses every two years:

$$\frac{20 \text{ years}}{2 \text{ years}} = 10 \text{ pairs of glasses}$$

Therefore, 10 pairs of glasses X $200 = $2000

Daily wear contact lenses:

$200

Assume you change your lenses every 18 months:

$$\frac{20 \text{ years}}{18 \text{ months}} = 13 \text{ pairs of contact lenses}$$

Therefore, 13 pairs of lenses X $200 = $2600

Disposable contact lenses:

$300 per year

Assume you change your lenses every two weeks:

Therefore, $300 per year X 20 years = $6000

Taking into account a compound interest rate of 6%, the final costs are as follows (prices below represent an approximate typical cost in 1997 U.S. dollars for *both* eyes.):

Glasses	**$1300**
Daily wear contact lenses	**$1600**
Disposable contact lenses	**$3500**

Compare these numbers with the surgical fees quoted for your procedure of choice.

TAX

As always, ignoring the whole question of taxation is probably not a good idea. Although the details depend on your region and income bracket, refractive surgery may be tax deductible. It would be a good idea to check with your accountant who, if the stereotypes are correct, has considerable experience with both money and glasses. When tax is factored into the equation, refractive surgery may appear to be more cost-effective than at first glance.

13

THE PATIENTS' PERSPECTIVE

They made the decision, took the plunge, and lived to tell about it. Who better than to ask about laser eye surgery than the patients themselves?

PRK - A Patient's Perspective,
By Janet Taylor

It has been called vision sculpting, laser sight enhancement, and the wave of the future. It is photorefractive keratectomy and my decision to go ahead with this miraculous surgery was not a frivolous one. I started my research into PRK in 1991. At the time, the procedure was new to my area and the ads seemed too good to be true. Was it really possible to see clearly without glasses or contact lenses?

I began wearing glasses when I was in grade seven. They were fine for school, but when it came to sports, I found that they were cumbersome and somewhat dangerous. I tried my first pair of contact lenses two years later, but they were never quite right for me. I was never really comfortable in contact lenses and

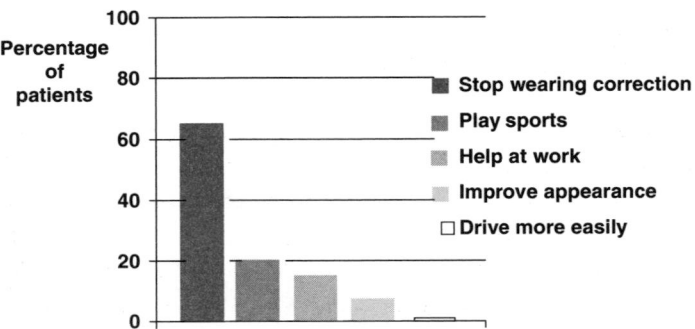

PRK
Why Did You Decide to Have
the Treatment?

Percentage of patients

- Stop wearing correction
- Play sports
- Help at work
- Improve appearance
- Drive more easily

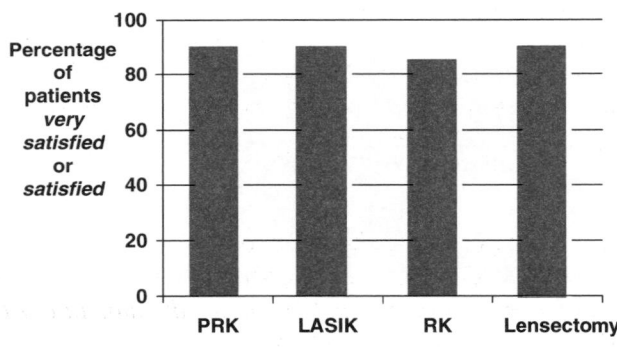

Patient Satisfaction

Percentage of patients *very satisfied* or *satisfied*

PRK   LASIK   RK   Lensectomy

because my eyes are dry, I was usually ready to remove them after only a few hours of wear. Also, I found the cleaning solutions to be a bother. There were too many steps and it took far too long to clean the lenses. Eventually, I found myself wearing the lenses for only special occasions. Naturally, when the idea of not having to wear contact lenses or glasses was suggested to me, I was interested, but somewhat skeptical.

I gathered as much information as I could find on PRK and other kinds of refractive surgery. During the time when I was pursuing the idea of having laser eye surgery, my friends and family were continually cautioning me against the procedure. I heard comments like, "it's too new", "it's still experimental", and "what if you go blind?". I was frightened by their remarks and I persevered with my glasses for almost four more years.

I finally gathered enough courage, and on December 13, 1995 (even though 13 is supposed to be unlucky), I underwent PRK on my left eye. The experience was a memorable one. A week before the surgery, I had my eyes examined by the surgeon with whom I had consulted three years earlier. I was nervous and I thought I might still back out of my decision. My family was not aware that I was having PRK, and on the day of the procedure, I arrived at the laser centre alone. The surgeon examined my eyes again, and reviewed the benefits and risks. I was asked to sign a consent form. I was then taken to an area to have drops inserted into my eye. I was told that the purpose of the drops was to prevent infection and to freeze my eye. As the drops were applied, I could feel my heart beat a little faster and I began to break out in a cold sweat. But being a very chatty person, I just kept talking to the staff and that helped to ease my nerves.

After three sets of drops, I was led into the laser room. I sat down in a chair similar to that in a dentist's office. Once the chair had moved back into a reclining position, the technician positioned me under the machine. At that point, I knew that there was no turning back! I was asked to stare at a red light, which was a rather difficult task. My eye was watering and I felt a heavy sensation. The surgeon used an instrument to hold my eyelids back and prevent me from blinking during the procedure. I was given more drops and we were "ready to go"! I heard the laser whir and there were three soft clicks - SLAP, SLAP, SLAP. I felt nothing except for the beating of my racing heart. I did notice a funny smell, but I was too busy trying to focus on the red light to really pay attention to anything else. After about ten seconds, the surgeon turned the light brighter, while I continued to focus on the red light which

PRK
How Would You Describe Your Feelings
About the Treatment?

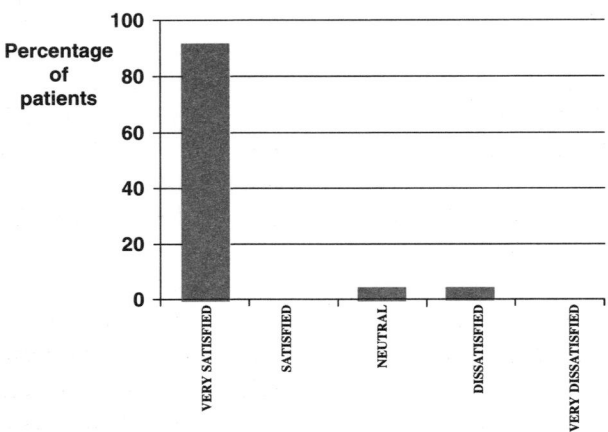

PRK
Have You Noticed Any Benefits in Your Work,
Home, or Social Life?

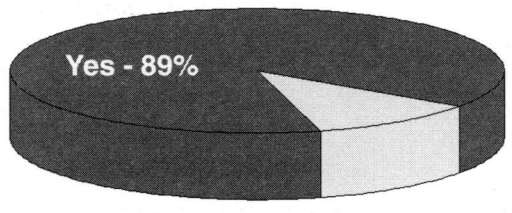

was, by then, only a red blur. At that point, I remember thinking thoughts like "it isn't working" and "why am I doing this?".

As the procedure continued, I saw a kaleidoscope of lights. I heard the surgeon say that he was smoothing the surface and I noticed my vision getting even blurrier. Then, I was told that "this time is for real". I was instructed to stare at the red light, which was almost impossible with such blurry vision. The technician kept cheering me on and guiding me to keep my fixation. This time, the whir of the laser was quieter. I heard the same three soft clicks and "blip, blip" as the laser worked. I noticed my vision changing and red light came in and our of focus during the twenty seconds or so which constituted the first part of my treatment.

After a short break, during which I resisted the urge to blink, the second phase of the procedure began. I heard the same noises as before and I noticed the red light as it seemed to move. I was afraid that I might have been moving my eye but the reassurances of the technician indicated that I was fixating properly. The procedure was over in seconds, even if it did seem like an eternity! The surgeon put a contact lens in my eye to act as a bandage and (of course!) more drops. As I sat up, I noticed that things were brighter and I could define some images quite well.

I was taken to another room to have my eye examined and I was given instructions and some eye drops to apply over the next few days. That night, I went out for dinner with a friend, and to my surprise, my eye was not hurting at all. The following morning, I felt a scratchy sensation when I awoke. After I applied the drops, I felt better. I then attended a conference, which I had registered for several months earlier. Although I found that bright lights made me uncomfortable. I was determined to persevere, and I made it through the meeting with little difficulty.

In the afternoon, I had an appointment with my surgeon. He said that my vision was improving, but slowly. I was anxious, but positive. On the third day, I was supposed to have the contact lens out, but the surgeon decided to wait because my epithelium had not completely healed. I was not sure how to take this news, but because I trusted my surgeon, I decided not to worry. By the end of the week, the lens was removed and I was able to read the 20/30 line. Even though that was supposed to be good, I wasn't really happy. I wanted perfection! (Doesn't everybody?) It took at least a month until I could read the 20/20 line with ease. Then I was ecstatic! It was really worth waiting

PRK
Where Have You Noticed the Benefits?

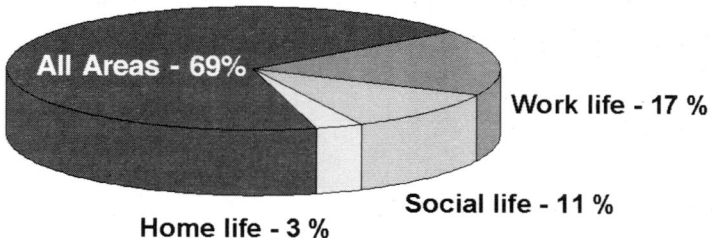

Home life - 3 %

PRK
Would You Recommend This Treatment to a Friend?

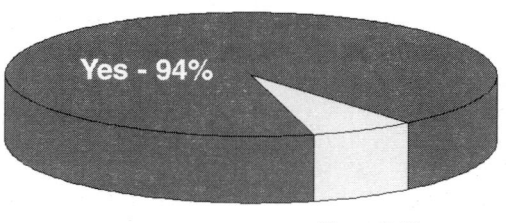

No - 6 %

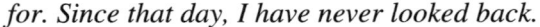

for. Since that day, I have never looked back.

I am very happy with the results of the laser surgery. Although I recognize that surgery should never be entered into without careful consideration of the risks involved, I am certainly glad that I did it. I am also glad that I was so fully prepared. I think that education is the key to preparation. The more you know about the procedure, the better prepared you will be.

PRK - A Doctor's Perspective,
By Richard Lewis M.D.

The excitement of refractive surgery was present for me both professionally and personally. I have been an ophthalmologist since 1979, but I had been myopic since I was a teenager. I was able to wear contact lenses until I entered medical school. There, I developed contact lens related allergies with uncomfortable, irritated, often red eyes. Glasses were the only option for me until refractive surgery became available. Eyeglasses were satisfactory for work, but not during my recreation and hobbies. Skiing, golf, tennis, and other sports were difficult in wet or misty conditions.

I was able to witness the progression of refractive surgery from the initial trials involving refractive keratotomy. Problems that became evident with RK, including fluctuating vision, progressive hyperopia, and varying surgical techniques discouraged me from performing this surgery as well as personally undergoing the procedure. So much is dependent on my acuity and binocular vision (or stereopsis) for my professional career that I wanted to wait until a more precise and predictable procedure became available. I remained a very interested observer in this developing specialty, though very reluctant to proceed.

Photorefractive surgery was first popularized over the last six years. During 1994, a number of my patients and colleagues, including my partner, travelled to Canada to have the procedure. As I had the opportunity to examine him during the post-operative recovery, I became aware of the safety and effectiveness of the procedure.

RK
Would You Recommend This Treatment to a Friend?

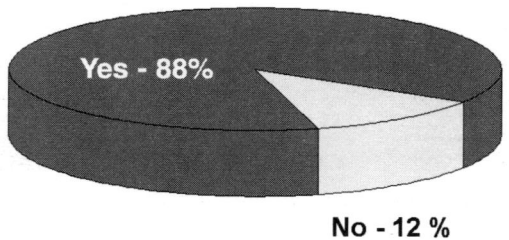

Yes - 88%

No - 12 %

PRK
Would You Have Your Second Eye Treated?
(For Those Who Have Had Only One Eye Treated)

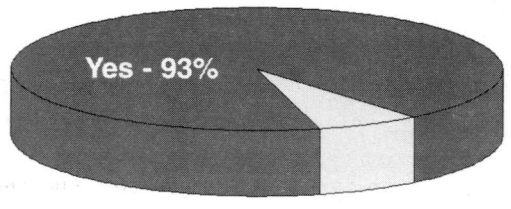

Yes - 93%

No - 7 %

I decided to personally undergo the surgery late in 1995. I investigated various ophthalmic surgeons who performed the procedure. At that time, it was not approved in the United States. I elected to have it completed by a surgeon who had extensive experience and one whom I had known and trusted for many years. Once this decision was reached, like so many patients, I wanted to do it as soon as possible and have both eyes operated on at the same sitting. As an ophthalmologist, I was quite aware that surgery on both eyes simultaneously is rarely recommended with concern about infections and other complications. My research in PRK indicated that these concerns, though possible, were very rare. Also, there is one other advantage in simultaneous, bilateral surgery, and it has to do with recovery. I recognized that I would be unable to return to work for about one week. Undergoing the surgery in both eyes would keep this and the period of post-operative glare to a minimum.

The PRK surgery was successfully completed in both eyes during the week of Thanksgiving. As I expected, I had glare and some discomfort for the first four days. I used eye drops to prevent infection and enhance healing but did not require pain medications. After 48 hours, I tried to return to work. I had some initial problems with visual blurring and glare, and was unable to return to my full duties for seven days.

The first post-operative month was characterized by a subtle change in vision, especially in contrast. This was evident when looking at certain colors and fine detail, such as newsprint. I was slightly farsighted in the beginning, creating a slight blur for near objects. Other visual tasks, such as those in surgery or in recreation, were not impeded during this period. My vision returned to 20/20 four weeks after surgery and has remained at this level ever since.

It was interesting trying to adapt to life without glasses. I was not accustomed to seeing so clearly while taking a shower. For weeks, I would reach up, assuming that I had forgotten to take my glasses off, only to be surprised that they were not there. It was a very pleasant surprise to be able to watch television without glasses. It has been wonderful participating in outdoor sports, especially water sports or skiing. For the first time, I was able to see exotic fish while snorkelling. In fact, all of the inconveniences during recreation that provoked the surgery in the first place, are no longer a problem.

In surgical consultations, patients often ask me if I would recommend the proposed procedure to my family. In the case of refractive surgery with PRK, I have been so satisfied with my personal results that I wholeheartedly reply, "Yes".

Refractive lensectomy - A Doctor's Perspective,
By Angus MacDonald M.D.

I received my first glasses at the age of six. Like all lifelong myopes, I yearned for better uncorrected visual acuity, for cosmetic, recreational, and occupational reasons. In addition, I wanted to rid myself of the underlying, almost subconscious feeling of weakness associated with being almost (in fact, legally) blind without glasses or contact lenses. Compounding this was the fact that I turned out to be contact lens intolerant.

After a great deal of thought, I decided to pursue refractive surgery. I explored the alternatives of PRK and LASIK, and decided to undergo refractive lensectomy. My decision was based on several factors. Being over the age of 50, my presbyopic crystalline lens was not much use for accommodation. My high myopia (-9.50 D) also tipped the scales in favor of lensectomy, as did my personal experience and confidence in the procedure itself. (As an ophthalmologist, I have found myself on the other end of the identical procedure on numerous occasions.) Not to be overlooked was my confidence in the surgeon. I had a lot to lose if the procedure was not performed flawlessly.

The procedure itself was performed under topical anaesthesia without sedation. The microscope light was very bright but I knew I had to maintain central fixation to facilitate my surgeon's operative view. Did it hurt? No. There was never any sharp pain, but there was a definite aching sensation as the phacoemulsification needle entered my eye and the anterior chamber was pressurized with fluid. This lasted about 30 seconds. I had a moment of, not panic, but emotional concern, when my own crystalline lens was completely removed. I felt blind. All I saw was total diffuse whiteness and no form. However, I knew what was happening and calmed myself down awaiting the most incredible experience that followed. I actually saw, albeit blurred, each component of the implant entering my eye.

I keep reliving this experience over and over. It was scary, thrilling, and life-changing for me. My only regret is that technology, my surgeon, and I didn't come together at an earlier date.

PART FIVE

THE DECISIONS

14

REFRACTIVE SURGERY: THE BIG QUESTIONS

IF?

Studies show that most people take between six months and a year to make the decision. It doesn't have to take that long.

Should I have refractive surgery? A self-test.

Instructions

1. Read the following statements. Put a check mark beside the ones which apply to you.
2. Highlight or underline the lines corresponding to these elected statements.
3. Add up the columns, counting only the highlighted or underlined eyes.
4. See which column has the greater number of total eyes. The eyes have it.
5. A *bomb*, when highlighted, means that this alternative is inappropriate for you.
6. This is to be used as a guide only. The final decision should be made by you and your doctor.

	Yes	No
About you		
I am under 18	💣	▪
I am not financially stable and have no means to pay for elective surgery	💣	▪
I have serious active medical illness	💣	▪
I adapt easily to change	👁 👁	▪
I am a perfectionist and little irregularities bother me	▪	👁 👁
My appearance is very important to me	👁	▪
I am an anxious, nervous person	▪	👁
I believe that a one in a thousand risk could never happen to me	▪	👁 👁
I believe that nothing in life is risk free	👁 👁	▪
I can tolerate short-term pain for long-term gain	👁	▪
The main reason for having surgery is that my spouse/boyfriend/girlfriend wants me to	▪	👁 👁 👁
Subtotal 1	_____	_____

About your eyes	Yes	No
I have only one good eye	💣	—
I have significant eye disease	💣	—
My refractive error has been unstable in the last year	💣	—
I am mildly myopic	👁👁👁	—
I am moderately myopic	👁👁	—
I am severely myopic	👁	—
I am mildly hyperopic	👁👁👁	—
I am moderately hyperopic	👁👁	—
I am severely hyperopic	👁	—
I have perfect vision with glasses or contact lenses	—	👁
I have no difficulty with contact lenses	—	👁👁👁
I have never attempted to wear contact lenses	—	👁👁

Subtotal 2   _____   _____

	Yes	No
I am unable to wear contact lenses	👁👁👁	▬
I believe that anything less than 20/20 post-operatively would be disappointing	▬	👁👁
I have a good reason for wanting refractive surgery	👁👁👁	▬
My refractive error interferes with my occupation	👁👁👁	▬
My refractive error interferes with my recreation	👁👁👁	▬
My refractive error does not bother me	▬	👁👁👁
I would consider surgery a success if my uncorrected vision is improved, even if it isn't perfect	👁👁	▬
I fear being incapacitated if I should ever lose my glasses or contacts	👁👁👁	▬

Subtotal 3	_____	_____
Subtotal 2	_____	_____
Subtotal 1	_____	_____
__Total__	_____	_____

WHEN?

You may have already decided to have laser eye surgery. The big question is when. Now or later? The psychic hotlines aside, nobody can predict the future. Tomorrow, they may invent a two dollar pill that cures myopia. Doubtful, but who would have imagined PRK twenty years ago. So it is a personal decision, to wait or not to wait. To help crystallize your thoughts, it may be a good idea to ask yourself, "What am I waiting for?"

What am I waiting for? A self-test.

Instructions
1. Put a check mark, in the "before column", beside the statements that apply to you.
2. For each one you have chosen, read the corresponding paragraph. After you have read the section, try to decide if your chosen statements still make sense.
3. If they do, place a check mark beside the appropriate statements in the "after" column.
4. If there are one or more "after" responses checked, that means that you have a good reason to wait. So wait.
5. This is to be used as a guide only. The final decision should be made by you and your doctor.

Before   **After**

_____   I'm waiting for the cost to come down.   _____

_____   I'm waiting for long-term safety to be established.   _____

_____   I'm waiting for techniques and equipment to improve.   _____

_____   I'm waiting for results to improve.   _____

_____   I'm waiting for my surgeon to become more experienced.   _____

_____   I'm waiting for the debate between PRK and LASIK to be resolved.   _____

Before		After
____	**I'm waiting for FDA approval.**	___
____	**I'm waiting for painless surgery.**	___
____	**I'm waiting until I can afford it.**	___
____	**I'm waiting until my insurance covers it.**	___
____	**I'm waiting because I'm scared.**	___

I'm waiting for the cost to come down: Fair enough. By how much? Depending on how much you want to pay, you may be waiting a while (see Chapter 12). It may be helpful to think about specific numbers. If the cost drops below two thousand for both eyes, would you do it. Or two hundred. Whatever. If you find yourself at a buck an eye and still wavering, then maybe cost isn't the rate limiting factor.

I'm waiting for long-term safety to be established: Good point. Tomorrow, they may find that PRK causes your hair to turn red. Unlikely, but who foresaw the problem with breast implants. It comes down to personal preference, risk tolerance, and the level of dissatisfaction with your current visual situation. If long-term results are important to you, you must define long-term. Twenty years? In order to know for certain that PRK has no detrimental effects on the eye twenty years after the procedure, patients must be followed for, well, twenty years. Doing a little math, if the first human studies were done in 1987, then you'll have your answer around the year 2007. For fifty year data, give yourself another thirty years or so. How long can you wait? That's up to you. If you can wait forever, then wait forever. Evidently your eyes are not bothering you very much right now so why rock the boat. If long term safety is the limiting factor, and you can't wait forever, then figure out how long you can wait. And wait.

I'm waiting for techniques and equipment to improve: Sounds reasonable. Techniques and equipment are improving every day. But what is your endpoint? It is not unlike buying a computer. Things are changing so rapidly, a new computer is almost out of date by the time you have everything connected. A state of the art 386 seemed like a good investment at the time, but now you can buy a fully loaded high end Pentium for a fraction of the cost. Not only that, three years from now, the new Octium (or whatever) will make you question your 1997 sanity. Does that mean you shouldn't buy now? Or that you shouldn't have bought that 386? Did you get any use out of that old model in the last few years? Was it worth it? With computers and with refractive surgery, you can wait forever for the next big thing. If you want to jump in, sooner or later, you'll have to pick a spot.

I'm waiting for results to improve: Results, too, are improving every day. Assume you have a 90% chance of achieving 20/20 uncorrected. You're waiting because that's not good enough. You should decide, then, what is good enough. 95%? 99%? 99.9%? If you believe that you're a one in a million kind of person who needs a success rate of 99.9999% to feel confident about surgery, then put on your glasses and wait. But know what you're waiting for.

I'm waiting for my surgeon to become more experienced: This is one life situation where it may not be best to be #1. There is a learning curve in performing laser eye surgery, but where do you draw the line? 10? 100? 1000? Is a surgeon who has performed 10,000 procedures better than someone who has done a paltry 1000? It depends on your level of concern. However, if you're waiting to be someone's one millionth customer, you'd better keep a lookout for a retirement party.

I'm waiting for the debate between PRK and LASIK to be resolved: Those of you with an old VCR in the basement may remember the Beta versus VHS dilemma. You'll be forgiven for drawing parallels. The last thing you want is obsolete eye surgery. That is, unless it works. If you have all the movies you'd ever want to watch sitting on your shelf in full Betamax glory, who cares about VHS? If you can see 20/20 uncorrected after PRK, or even RK, who cares about this whole LASIK thing? There's no harm in waiting until there is a consensus opinion, however that may take a few years. The question here is, will the wait be worth it?

I'm waiting for FDA approval: That bouncer at the door can be moody. You may be waiting a while. That's fine, if FDA approval gives you some sense of security and you're in no rush. The job of the FDA is to protect you from harm and there is something to be said for their stamp of approval. Nonetheless, there are those who feel that the FDA can be overprotective. Compounding the problem is that the FDA is considering hardball software modification to prevent "off-label" use of approved lasers. Bear in mind that there are people across the U.S. who are having surgery which has not been approved by the FDA. In the name of experimentation, thousands of informed volunteers have already had LASIK. Across the Canadian border, LASIK is being done without batting an eyelid. That may or may not be good enough for you. If it isn't, wait for FDA approval. But if you know the car you want and you know how to get it, what are you waiting for?

I'm waiting for painless surgery: Nobody likes pain. There is less pain with today's techniques than with earlier surgery. Especially with LASIK, the chance of significant pain is pretty low. If you're waiting for the incidence and severity of post-operative pain to drop even further, that is a real possibility, with better techniques and drugs. If you're waiting until there is zero chance of any pain, your surgery should probably be performed at Fantasyworld General Hospital.

I'm waiting until I can afford it: Everybody, with the exception of professional athletes, has limited resources. It is a question of priorities. If the choice is between buying food or having refractive surgery, perhaps lunch should take precedence. Most of the time, however, the decision is a little more difficult. A vacation, a new sound system, or a computer all vie for your discretionary dollar. Everybody has their own priorities. Make your list and if refractive surgery is not at the top, wait until it is.

I'm waiting until my insurance covers it: Don't hold your breath. Health care is in a disarray even without refractive surgery. American insurance companies are kicking new mothers out of the hospital two days after delivery. In Canada, the government can no longer always afford even life-saving treatments. The majority of prospective patients state that the number one deterrent to having laser eye surgery is the cost. What do you think would happen to the health care system if it were to suddenly cover an elective procedure such as refractive surgery? The entire network would be overwhelmed and destroyed. Even if the next American president is a contact lens intolerant -5 D myopic athlete, it is a difficult scenario to envision.

I'm waiting because I'm scared: Scared of what? The chance of something going wrong? Pain? Complications? What's probably scaring you is, no matter what you call it, the risk. There are risks involved in refractive surgery. And there will always be risks. And there will always be benefits. It is up to you to examine that risk/benefit ratio and make the decision. If you decide to wait, that's fine. Realize that you are waiting for that ratio to change. And probably, the potential benefits will remain the same as time goes by. So you're really waiting for the risks to drop. The question is, to what? Zero equals never. Being scared of the risks is natural. Wait until you're comfortable with the risks and benefits of refractive surgery.

WHICH DOCTOR?

Before you pull out your checkbook, make sure that you are happy with your choice of doctor.

> Is this the right doctor for me? A self-test.

Instructions
1. **Read the following statements.**
2. **Check either the yes or no box.**
3. **If there are one or more "no" responses, these issues should be addressed pre-operatively.**

	Yes	No
I have met the surgeon.	——	——
I am impressed with his or her qualifications and experience.	——	——
I am comfortable with his or her bedside manner.	——	——
All of my questions have been answered satisfactorily.	——	——
The facilities appear clean and modern.	——	——
The support staff are well-trained and helpful.	——	——
I am satisfied with the planned post-operative care.	——	——
Someone is available should problems occur.	——	——

WHICH PROCEDURE?

Suppose you have decided that you should have refractive surgery, and that the time is now. The next question is which procedure you should select.

> The Myope: Which procedure is best for me? A self-test.

Instructions

1. Read the following statements. Put a check mark beside the ones which apply to you.
2. Highlight or underline the lines corresponding to these selected statements.
3. Add up the columns, counting only the highlighted or underlined eyes.
4. See which column has the greater number of total eyes. The eyes have it.
5. A *bomb*, when highlighted, means that this alternative is inappropriate for you.
6. A *star* represents the ideal alternative
7. This is to be used as a guide only. The final decision should be made by you and your doctor.

About you	LASIK	PRK	RK	Lensectomy
I am over 50 years old	👁	👁	👁	👁👁👁
I am between 40 and 50 years old	👁	👁	👁	👁👁
I am under 40 years old	👁	👁	👁	—
Subtotal 1	___	___	___	___

	LASIK	PRK	RK	Lensectomy
I would prefer to sacrifice a little comfort for safety	👁	👁👁👁	👁	👁
It is important to me to know that the long-term safety has been proven	–	👁	👁👁	👁👁👁
I believe in technology	👁👁👁	👁👁👁	–	👁
I do not trust computers	–	–	👁👁👁	👁
I have great difficulty using eye drops	👁👁	💣	👁👁	👁
I have been told I have impaired wound healing	👁👁👁	👁	👁	👁👁

About your eyes

	LASIK	PRK	RK	Lensectomy
I am mildly myopic (-1 D to -3 D)	👁	👁👁👁	👁👁👁	👁

Subtotal 2   ____   ____   ____   ____

	LASIK	PRK	RK	Lensectomy
I am moderately myopic (-3.25 D to -6 D)	2 eyes	3 eyes	–	2 eyes
I am severely myopic (-6.25 D to -9 D)	3 eyes	1 eye	1 eye	3 eyes
I have already had RK	1 eye	2 eyes	–	2 eyes
I would like to have both eyes operated on together	3 eyes	2 eyes	2 eyes	1 eye
I have changes in my crystalline lens	–	–	–	★
Speed of recovery is very important to me	3 eyes	1 eye	2 eyes	2 eyes
Pain is a very important factor to me	3 eyes	1 eye	2 eyes	2 eyes
I would hate having to undergo a retreatment	2 eyes	2 eyes	1 eye	3 eyes

Subtotal 3   ___   ___   ___   ___

	LASIK	PRK	RK	Lensectomy
I would like to retain the ability to focus up close (accommodate)	👁	👁	👁	💣
My eyes respond poorly to steroids	👁👁👁	💣	👁👁👁	👁
Subtotal 4	___	___	___	___
Subtotal 3	___	___	___	___
Subtotal 2	___	___	___	___
Subtotal 1	___	___	___	___
___Total___	___	___	___	___

The Hyperope: Which procedure is best for me? A self-test.

Instructions

1. Read the following statements. Put a check mark beside the ones which apply to you.
2. Highlight or underline the lines corresponding to these selected statements.
3. Add up the columns, counting only the highlighted or underlined eyes.
4. See which column has the greater number of total eyes. The eyes have it.
5. A *bomb*, when highlighted, means that this alternative is inappropriate for you.
6. A *star* represents the ideal alternative
7. This is to be used as a guide only. The final decision should be made by you and your doctor.

About you	HK	Lensectomy	LTK	PRK	LASIK
I am over 50 years old	—	3 eyes	—	—	—
I am between 40 and 50 years old	—	2 eyes	1 eye	1 eye	1 eye
I am less than 40 years old	1 eye	—	1 eye	1 eye	1 eye
Safety is my number one concern	—	1 eye	2 eyes	3 eyes	2 eyes
Long-term data is important to me	2 eyes	3 eyes	1 eye	1 eye	—
Subtotal 1	___	___	___	___	___

	HK	Lensectomy	LTK	PRK	LASIK
I believe in technology	–	👁👁	👁👁👁	👁👁👁	👁👁👁
I do not trust computers	👁👁👁	👁👁	–	–	–
I have great difficulty using eye drops	👁👁	👁	👁👁	–	👁👁
I have impaired wound healing	👁	👁👁	👁👁	👁	👁👁👁

About your eyes

	HK	Lensectomy	LTK	PRK	LASIK
I am mildly hyperopic (Plano to +3 D)	👁	👁	👁👁	👁👁	👁
I am moderately hyperopic (+3.25 to +6 D)	👁	👁👁	👁	👁👁	👁👁
I am severely hyperopic (+6.25 to +10 D)	–	👁👁👁	–	👁	👁👁
I have already had a refractive surgery	–	👁👁	👁	👁👁	👁👁

	HK	Lensectomy	LTK	PRK	LASIK
Subtotal 2	___	___	___	___	___

	HK	Lensectomy	LTK	PRK	LASIK
I have changes in my crystalline lens	-	★	-	-	-
Speed of recovery is important to me	👁👁	👁👁	👁👁	👁	👁👁
Pain is very important to me	👁👁	👁👁👁	👁👁👁	👁	👁👁
I would like to retain the ability to focus at near	-	💣	-	-	-
My eyes respond poorly to steroids	👁👁👁	👁	👁👁👁	💣	👁👁👁
Subtotal 3	___	___	___	___	___
Subtotal 2	___	___	___	___	___
Subtotal 1	___	___	___	___	___
Total	___	___	___	___	___

TWO EYES TOGETHER?

Now that you've decided to have surgery and you know which doctor is doing what procedure, there is one big question left.

Should I have surgery on both eyes at one time? A self test.

Instructions

1. **Read the following statements. Put a check mark beside the ones which apply to you.**
2. **Highlight or underline the lines corresponding to these selected statements.**
3. **Add up the columns, counting only the highlighted or underlined eyes.**
4. **See which column has the greater number of total eyes. The eyes have it.**
5. **This is to be used as a guide only. The final decision should be made by you and your doctor.**

	Yes	No
I plan to have LASIK	👁	▪
I plan to have PRK	▪	👁
I would rather get it all over with at once	👁	▪
The thought of blurred vision in both eyes is frightening to me	▪	👁
Subtotal 1	____	____

	Yes	No
The prospect of rare bilateral complications doesn't bother me	👁	▬
If the first eye doesn't go well, I wouldn't have the other one done	▬	👁
Safety is my number one priority	▬	👁
Convenience is my number one priority	👁	▬
I'm interested in monovision	▬	👁
There is somebody to help look after me post-operatively	👁	▬
FDA recommendations are important to me	▬	👁
Subtotal 2	___	___
Subtotal 1	___	___
Total	___	___

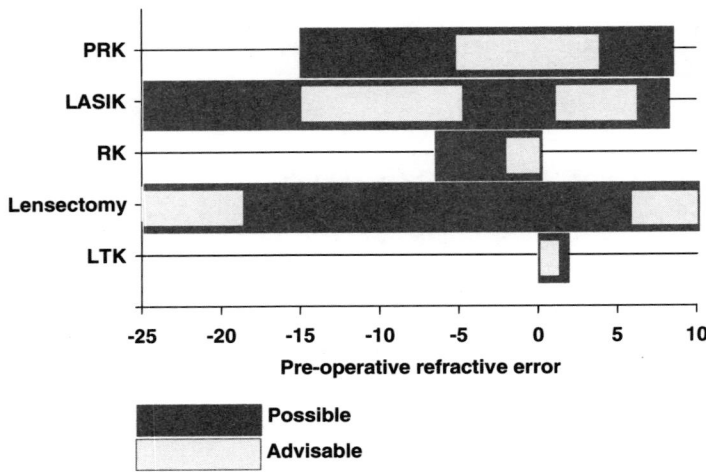

PART SIX

HINDSIGHT

List of Abbreviations

ACIOL	Anterior Chamber Intraocular Lens
AK	Astigmatic Keratotomy
ALK	Automated Lamellar Keratoplasty
CME	Cystoid Macular Edema
D	Diopter
D.O.	Doctor of Osteopathy
ICR	Intrastromal corneal ring
IOP	Intraocular pressure
F.A.A.O.	Fellow of the American Academy of Optometry
FDA	Food and Drug Administration
F.R.C.S(C.)	Fellow of the Royal College of Physicians and Surgeons of Canada
HK	Hexagonal Keratotomy
LASER	Light Amplification by Stimulated Emission of Radiation
LASIK	Laser In Situ Keratomileusis
M.D.	Doctor of Medicine
mm	millimetre
NSAID	Non-steroidal Anti-inflammatory Drug
O.D.	Doctor of Optometry
OD	Right eye
OS	Left eye
OU	Both eyes
PCIOL	Posterior Chamber Intraocular Lens
PRK	Photo Refractive Keratectomy
RK	Radial Keratotomy

Index